RIGHT WEIGHT, RIGHT MIND:

The ITC Approach to Permanent Weight Loss

...as featured in O: The Oprah Magazine

Dr. Robert Kegan, Dr. Lisa Lahey, and Dr. Deborah Helsing

Minds at Work, LLC
1208 Massachusetts Avenue, Suite 3
Cambridge, MA 02138
www.mindsatwork.com
617-491-2656

Table of Contents

INTRODUCTION

Building a Bridge

"Why do people say it's so hard to quit smoking? Hell, I've done it hundreds of times myself!"
– often attributed to Mark Twain

If you ask any group of people (as we have now done many times, in every part of the world), "raise your hand if you'd like to lose some weight," it is always the same—a majority of hands will instantly reach for the sky. Yet *losing* weight is actually not that hard. Most of those who raise their hands have lost weight, some of them many times. You, yourself, *have* lost weight, haven't you? Probably many times. The big uncracked problem with weight is not really about how to lose it—*but how to keep it off*. On average, dieters regain 107% of the weight they take off on a diet!

From Wanting to Change to Being Able to Change

Here is a note from one publisher we asked to consider this book:

> I've read your manuscript from cover to cover, and even tried out the map-making. Your approach might be the most powerful contribution to weight-loss I have seen in fifty years. But no one is going to use it because it is too hard. It takes a couple months for people to get their minds right. People don't care about their minds; they want to change their bodies. And they want it fast. People would rather buy a book that will give them a fast solution that doesn't work than a slower one that does.

This particular publisher went on to reject our manuscript.

To be clear: what you are reading right now is not a diet book. You don't need another diet book. There are plenty of great diets out there and if you follow them they will all help you lose weight. But none of them will really help you keep the weight off. We are not medical doctors. We are doctors of the mind—Harvard-trained, adult-developmental psychologists—and we have spent a generation working on just one problem: how do you help people make permanent changes, changes that last, changes that do not, after a while, leave you back where you started? Or worse off by 7%?

Now that, as Mark Twain knew, is a hard problem, a really hard problem. Recent studies show that doctors can tell their heart patients they will literally die if they do not permanently change their ways (concerning diet, smoking, exercise) and still only about one in seven will be able to make the changes. These are not people who want to die. They urgently want to live out their lives, fulfill their dreams, watch their grandchildren grow up—and still, they cannot make the changes they need to in order to survive.

If *wanting* to change and actually *being able* to change are so uncertainly linked when our very lives are on the line, why should we expect that we will be able to do any better when the stakes are even smaller—if losing weight, and keeping it off, is not for most of us a life-and-death matter?

The answer to this question, we discovered, is that being able to do what you intend is not primarily a matter of having a big enough pay-off, or a great enough sense of urgency. It is primarily about uncovering a hidden mechanism in your mind, which this book will teach you about. Once you uncover it—and can make concrete, practical use of it—you will be able to build a bridge from ***What You Want to Do to What You Can Do***, and you will be able to cross this bridge as often as you like.

We know this is true because we have taught this method to thousands of people all over the world, and have heard from or *personally* seen hundreds of them achieve their desired results in a matter of months by practicing what they have learned. And we find that once they shift their focus from "right behavior" to "right mind," the changes they seek in their behavior (eating differently, for example) *persist*. They don't disappear a year later.

You will meet lots of real people in this book, people who courageously took the journey you are about to undertake. We hope these stories provide both insights and a chorus of support for your efforts. Let's start with a story that's very close to home.

A Personal Odyssey

This is Bob Kegan now, speaking to you in the first person. Let me tell you a little story that is as embarrassing as it is true. If I were being completely honest, I'd tell you that for most of the last thirty years some part of my energy and attention had been unproductively caught up with my weight. I say "unproductively" because, although for much of this time I may have been OK with my weight, I *never* had the feeling I wasn't "fighting." I may have had "winning periods," but I always felt I was in a kind of battle.

I would slowly get to a weight I didn't like—clothes too tight, not liking how I looked in the mirror or in photos—and I would then "successfully diet." I would take off the weight, enjoy how I felt and looked, and remind myself not to put it back on too quickly. And I *didn't* put it back on too quickly. But inevitably I did put it back on.

Now that is not the embarrassing part. A few years ago I decided I had had enough of all the time "contending" with this weight thing. I wanted to be free of it. I stopped weighing myself. I stopped thinking too much about what and how and when I was eating. I just ate what I enjoyed. I was less consistent with my exercise, too, because I happen to not like exercise for its own sake, so if I didn't feel like it I didn't.

For many months I was, for the first time in my adult life, happily free of this whole battle of the bulge. And then a funny thing happened. I woke up and realized I bulged. I mean I really bulged. I could hardly fit into any of my clothes. I got on a scale and discovered I was heavier than I had EVER been in my entire life. I had to put aside a significant portion of my wardrobe. I would calculate before a work trip whether I had enough trousers to pack that I could fit into. I'd look at clothes in my closet I enjoyed wearing and think, "I will never wear these again. That was a different era in my life."

I had been enjoying my freedom from thinking about weight and didn't want to give it up. Thankfully, I then happened upon yet another brilliant solution, which would allow me to continue "not contending." I went out and bought a few pairs of pants two sizes bigger than I had been wearing for years. Nice pants, fabrics I liked. "Why didn't I think of this sooner?" I asked myself. "There is a whole other, simpler route to fitting comfortably into your clothes, and not having that too-tight, over-stuffed feeling—just get bigger pants!"

With this stunningly inventive line of thinking and behavior I was on track to be 250 pounds and at risk for about a dozen chronic diseases. I'm not sure what really got me to thinking, "You are out of your mind. You have got to do *something* about this." I remember trying on half a dozen pairs of pants from my closet and *not even being able to zip them up!* A dear friend said, "You have got to lose that weight you are carrying around." I decided to do something.

Now, up to this point you are just hearing a version of every dieter's story. We hit some kind of bottom and decide to do something. We get resolve. We come up with a plan; we are full of passion, purpose, and sincerity. We change our ways, the weight begins to fall off, and people start telling us how good we look. We feel we have turned a corner. This is what we call "the New Year's Resolution approach to change." You know how this story ends. We *do* turn a corner—and we run smack into our old selves, which unfortunately have *not* changed. Our behavior has changed, but not our mind, and before we know it we have regained the weight.

But this story has a different ending. It was co-author Lisa Lahey who strongly urged me not to just do my normal diet. "Practice what you preach. Find out your own immunity on this, and make it part of your diet." You will soon enough learn what it means to follow Lisa's advice in practice (whether you are at the start of a diet, or have already lost the weight and this time you want to keep it off), but let me just fast-forward to tell you how things have come out for me:

- I didn't just lose the weight; I have—now several years later—kept it off.
- I have a completely different take on the whole food/weight situation.
- For the first time in my life, I am no longer "fighting" anything related to food and diet. The pleasure in being free of what I now realize I assumed was a life sentence is enormous.
- I no longer see maintaining a healthy, "right" weight as having anything to do with greater willpower, or becoming more disciplined, or making do with less. I do not see it as curbing my appetite. I do not feel deprived.
- On the contrary, my love of food is just as strong, and my sense of abundance in relation to eating is greater today than at any other time in my life.

From Professional to Personal: Our Work on Creating Permanent Change

So how did I get to this different result— a result we hear about regularly from people who have tried our approach? As we said, we spent a generation working to solve just one problem—how to help people make permanent change in areas that have resisted their smartest plans and their most heartfelt intentions. In the process we made an exciting discovery we are soon going to share with you. Initially, we only brought our approach to the world of work, including leadership development, work improvement, and higher performance among top teams. We have helped corporate executives and public-sector managers make the changes necessary for them to succeed in their jobs, changes they had tried to make in the past with only *temporary* success—just like dieters. We helped them to be braver communicators or to step out of the spotlight (and help others step into it). We helped them be better delegators, or better organized, or better with conflict. We helped them get closer to people, or worry less what people thought of them. Our approach to helping people make *lasting* change has now been adopted by a European railway, a state's Child Welfare office, an international strategy-consulting firm, one of the world's largest breweries, a leading pharmaceutical company, a school system, a telephone company, a hospital, a chain of movie theaters, and the U.S. Forest Service.

So now perhaps you are thinking, "This is a strange set of credentials for people suggesting they have the answer to sustainable weight-loss." We agree.

But something unexpected happened as our discovery took hold in the world of work: people began to try it out in their personal lives. Our ideas and practices began to migrate from the boardroom to the bedroom, from the conference table to the dinner table. People started to tell us they were using our work to change behaviors in their personal life they had tried for years to change without lasting success. "This worked for me where therapy did not—and lots faster," was a frequent message we received.

The most common focus people applied our work to in their personal lives was their weight. In 2010, *O: The Oprah Magazine* featured our work in the flagship January issue, and at the start of 2011 her website published a Top Ten list of "Things to Do to Get Fit in 2011." *Number One* on her list was to try out our "immunity to change (ITC) approach."

For the past several years we have been systematically pursuing the value of our approach towards helping people make changes in their personal lives, especially as they relate to health. Why don't people stay on "maintenance medications" that have no negative side effects, are covered by their insurance, and known to be necessary to avoid serious illness or death when they say they *want* to stay on them? Why don't people exercise regularly even when they vow to do so, and know it will add years to their lives? And why can't people eat without regaining a pound they took off on a diet when putting the weight back on is the very *last* thing they want to do?

Seeing Your Own Reality

Buddhas don't wash away sins with water,
Or heal suffering with laying on of hands,
Or transmit understanding into the minds of others.
They introduce beings to freedom
Through showing them reality.

-Matercheta in Buddhism for Busy People

Don't worry; we know we are not Buddhas, and don't pretend to be! But having worked now with many people whose change goals concern their weight and their relationship to food, these words resonate with us in two ways. First, we see and feel the *suffering* this subject has for so many people; we see the terrible guilt (or "sinfulness") people feel, when they have vowed, for example, not to eat that chocolate cake and find themselves raiding the refrigerator after the others have gone to bed. We see the way people feel enslaved by their own appetites and desire.

The other way these words speak to us is in their suggestion of how we can free ourselves from this ordinary suffering: a mirror. This book offers no magic wands or water. Instead, what we offer *is a better mirror* to show you a reality about yourself you need have no fear or shame to look at. We will teach you how to use the power of observation, data gathering, and analysis to help you get from where you are to where you want to be.

The reality we want to show you is more a strength you possess than a weakness that enslaves you. The strength you possess is that, more than you know, you will go to any length to protect what is most dear to you; you will even risk your life to do so. Better understanding this strength will enable you to move across the bridge from ***What You Want to Do*** to ***What You Can Do***.

What do we mean? A woman contacted us not long ago to tell us she had been battling her weight all of her life. "I'd be thirty pounds overweight, go on diets, lose the weight, only to pretty quickly regain it. Never keeping it off was terribly discouraging. My doctor told me this constant yo-yoing of weight loss and regain was almost as unhealthy as staying heavy. Either way, I was making myself miserable and looking at a bad future."

Why was she contacting us? "I just want you to know, I had tried everything you can imagine—diets, therapy, exercise, prayer. I even had my stomach stapled. Nothing worked for long. I looked at your approach and my first thought was, 'This looks hard. This looks harder than not eating or exercising.' But I could see it was a different kind of hard. And I could see that nothing else had worked. So I gave it a try. I lost thirty pounds—more than a year ago! The weight is gone, and it hasn't come back. And I know it is because of this immunity stuff. I just wanted to thank you. And if you ever need to tell somebody's story, tell mine." So thank you, Ida Rose. We will, and here it is.

Uncovering Hidden Commitments

The first thing our approach does is have you draw a full picture of all the ways *you* work against your own goal, how you undermine your sincere, even urgent, desire to accomplish your goal. Ida Rose made a fearless, honest list:

- I tell myself not to even bring certain foods into the house because they will just create temptation, but I buy them all the same. I buy small packages, but lots of them.
- I tell myself when I go out to eat that I will divide the serving in half, and set aside half, and I do. And then I finish my half, and eat the other half, too.
- I join exercise groups at my fitness center and then don't go.
- I make rules—nothing to eat after 9pm, 8 glasses of water a day, no fried foods—and then I follow them for a while, and then I follow them intermittently, and then I don't follow them at all.
- I commend myself at 10 pm for having had a good day—got a lot of work done, and ate healthy all day. And then I reward myself with a hot fudge sundae.

The list goes on, but you get the idea. Ida Rose can now take a hard look at her goal, on the one hand ("I want to get to a healthy weight and stay there"), and at all her contrary behaviors on the other. Now you may think this is the "better mirror"; you may think this is the "reality" we want you to show yourself in order to set yourself free.

You would be wrong.

What Ida Rose had done so far is important, but it is only a foundation to hold *one end* of the bridge. In order to build the foundation that will hold the other end—so there can *be* a bridge— Ida Rose had to uncover her *hidden* commitments. She knew she was committed to losing weight, and this was her real, urgent, and *visible* commitment. This is the commitment she had. But there are also commitments that *have her*! These are just as real, just as urgent, but *in*visible.

You will see in the pages ahead how we helped Ida Rose—and how we will help you, if you are willing—to make the invisible visible. Here, in her own words, is what she saw when she did:

> You don't say it exactly like this, but what I got out of your process was that you were saying there must be something awful for me about having the weight off, and—no disrespect—but that seemed crazy to me. 'You have no idea how much I hate being fat,' I thought, 'what could be worse than that?'
>
> But I went through the process as you suggested, and I got to something in one day I didn't really get to in several months of therapy. For about six different reasons it's embarrassing for me to talk about this, but here it is in abbreviated form: Whenever I lost the weight, I felt good about it, sure. But I felt something else too, that I was not really looking at. Men would come on to me when I was thin, and I couldn't deal with this.

Ida Rose then courageously gave us a picture of damaging, violative relationships with men, beginning in her own home in her teens. Her present-day accomplishments and self-possession were clearly hard won by creating a safe distance between herself and those experiences. But what the process showed her was that her equanimity was also being preserved by maintaining a safe distance between herself as a successful professional, loving aunt, and dear friend, on the one hand, and herself as a vulnerable partner in an intimate relationship, on the other.

> Your approach showed me that, yes, I had a deep commitment to losing weight. But at the very same time there was a deep commitment that 'had me'— to *staying* overweight, to not attracting romantic attention, to not possibly being an object of desire in some man's mind.

> I had never considered it this way, but as soon as your exercise led me in this direction I knew instantly it was true, because there had always been a part of my experience over those years of losing and regaining weight I could never understand, and just ignored, and that was this: whenever I regained the weight, and would start hauling out my fat-girl clothes again, I'd feel ashamed and depressed. And I'd feel something else, too: relief! My big "Aha!" was as big as it was because, for the first time, I had a home for that feeling of relief. I got what it was about.

One Foot on the Gas Pedal, One on the Brakes

Now Ida Rose is beginning to see the bigger picture of "reality" that could set her free. She sees a picture of herself with one foot on the gas pedal ("I want to lose weight") and one foot on the brakes ("I want to protect myself from ever re-entering a world that leaves me feeling so enraged and unprotected"). She now sees a system that *must* produce the very behaviors that will prevent her from accomplishing her goal—and not out of her weakness, but out of her strength. Overeating is defeating her visible goal of losing weight, but it is also consistently, faithfully, brilliantly serving her once-invisible goal of protecting herself from a dangerous world!

We said a look into our "better mirror" will show you an extraordinary reserve of strength, your capacity to go to any length to protect what is most dear to you; strength so awesome you will even risk your life to do so. What is most dear to us all is our own survival—not in some selfish or willful sense, but as an unconscious, unwilled expression of our participation in the work of our species, as a thousands-of-years-old inheritance hard-wired into our brains. The rational, analytic, still-evolving contemporary part of Ida Rose's brain (her neo-cortex) knows that she is actually risking her health, even her life, by being so overweight. But the ancient, inherited, single-minded, watchful and care-taking part of her brain (the amygdala) sees Ida Rose becoming thin and registers the reddest of Threat Level Red. It goes to work to save her from that annihilative world of sexual intimacy and restores her to the safety of being overweight. Between the one part of her brain and the other we have the foundations to build the bridge that enables a person to move from ***What I Want to Do*** to ***What I Can Do***.

The Immune System of the Mind

Between the foot on the gas and the foot on the brake, Ida Rose can see a system that keeps anything from changing. We call this the mind's "immune system." We have learned that the mind, like the body, has an immune system—a beautiful, intelligent, ancient force of nature that works every minute of every day, beyond our awareness, with one purpose in mind—to protect us, to keep us alive.

Most of the time the immune system works perfectly, keeping us out of troubles we have no idea about. But once in a while, when it sees a danger that is not really there, it can itself become a source of trouble, the way an autoimmune attack on parts of your own body or the rejection of a transplanted organ can cause you trouble. Its false alarm—causing it to reject important material the system may need to thrive or recover—can put us in danger, even as it is trying to fulfill its mission to protect us. *What if your own inability to change the way you eat is directly related, not to your lack of willpower or discipline but to the workings of your beautiful, intelligent, ancient but sometimes misguided immune system?*

Now you might be thinking, "I get how this could be helpful to Ida Rose, but I have had a fortunate life. There are no past traumas or dramatic dangers lurking behind my inability to keep my hands off that extra helping of lasagna. It just tastes delicious; I get hungry and I lose my willpower. For goodness' sakes, don't you have something to help me increase my willpower? Isn't that a much more promising route to my succeeding with my goals around food?"

Well, fair enough, and you have really asked two questions. So here are the answers in opposite order.

First, you are right that "increasing your willpower" is one of the most popular approaches to losing weight and keeping it off. It is also true that willpower *can* be increased; we don't dispute that. But we have just suggested to you why increases in willpower will *not* lead you to accomplish your goal. If there is something like a mind's "immune system" then increases in willpower amount to "pressing harder" on the gas pedal. The engine will rev up. What else will happen? Without realizing you are doing it, you will also "press harder" on the brake. Net result: You *have* increased willpower, but the car still isn't going anywhere!

Second, we are *not* suggesting that the reason you can't resist the second helping of lasagna is because you had a traumatic past you are unaware of. We are only suggesting that when you honestly look into the reason you are likely to find a deeper motivation, not simply that you were hungry or that you know it will be delicious. You are going to find a hidden goal or commitment that surprises you. And following that surprise, you are going to see that this is a hidden strength at work, that this goal is a way you are protecting yourself and keeping yourself out of a danger you are probably not aware you feel. You don't see or feel it right now because your immune system is doing such a good job protecting you from it. The threat is invisible. But we know for sure some part of your mind feels it's there.

Why can we say this with such confidence? Because thousands of people, from every part of the world, have been "introduced to freedom" by seeing just this kind of reality. If there is anything we are sure of it is this: if you have an ancient, inherited part of your brain which does nothing all day but scan the environment for possible sources of your demise, physical or psychological, it is going to find *something* from which it feels the need to protect you. It is going to come up with something not just every month or year. It is going to come up with something many times every day! Anything that will make you feel your value is diminished; that could make your world feel less in your control, or more unfair, or less predictable; anything that threatens your relationships, how much the people important to you like you, respect you, feel you are living up to their expectations, or being faithful to the shared bonds that hold you; any of these things will create prospective dangers from which your immune system will try to protect you. We call this hidden mechanism your *immunity* to change—your ITC.

Your Immune System is Yours Alone

Even for those with the most loving family in the world, we guarantee you that your immune system has not been idle. Since you have mentioned lasagna, let's give you another example. A fellow came to us with the same appreciation as Ida Rose. "I've never been able to lose weight and keep it off until I used your approach. I'd be happy to tell you how it worked for me, but I don't think you are going to understand."

"Why won't I understand?" one of us replied.

"Because you don't look to me like you are Italian," Tony said.

"I'm not, but give me a try."

"Okay," said Tony. "I belong to a tribe of people I dearly love, and we have a weekly, multi-generational, multi-course eating extravaganza! The Sunday meal. In my family the mortal sin is not about missing Sunday Mass; it's missing Sunday dinner. You don't show up, you are disrespecting your elders."

"Okay, but it's not just about showing up. You have to *eat. Mangia*! Whenever I've tried to lose weight, I do OK until Sunday. But when I refuse one aunt's extra portion of this or another aunt's extra portion of that, you can't believe what happens. They say the most horrible things. 'Whatsamattta, Tony? You're not one of us anymore? You're too good to eat your own family's food?' and then my Ma will say, 'Tony, why are you giving your aunts *agita*? Be a good boy.'"

"It isn't even what they say. You should see the looks on their faces! They aren't just offering me more pasta. They are offering me *love*. I'm saying no to the pasta, and they look like I threw their love right back into their faces."

"Quit smiling! You see, you're not Italian, and that's why you aren't getting this, but you helped me figure out my, whatdoyoucallit?, my 'hidden commitment,' my foot on the brake. I overeat on Sundays because I am committed to not hurting my loving aunts, to not being hurt myself when they say the things they do. The minute I saw how smart my overeating was, that created a whole new space for me. I was free!"

But maybe your immune system has no connection to your family of origin at all. Maybe it feels linked more to your current reality. Your own "foot on the brake" can stem from any number of ways you have been unknowingly trying to protect yourself to maintain control, your sense of identity, the terms of your relationships, emotional safety, or self-esteem. Our brains are wired to detect any signs of danger and protect ourselves from it, and so there are many different ways we can be over-protecting ourselves and immune to change.

The Dieter's Downfall: Technical Fixes Can't Resolve Adaptive Challenges

By now you might be thinking, "Hmmm, maybe there is something to this. I see how the 'picture of reality' helped Ida Rose and Tony see something important. But I don't quite see yet how they get *un*stuck. One foot is still on the gas, and one on the brake. They may know now *why* the car isn't moving, but not *how* to get it moving."

Fair enough. If you are feeling this way, you are about ready to finish this Introduction and dive into the book. The "picture of reality" is more like a diagnosis (and we can help you to create yours in about an hour or so). It will create an insight, and that insight creates the bridge. But an insight isn't a "cure" and a bridge doesn't get you anywhere if you don't walk over it.

We don't want to end this introduction without a few words to help you make it from one end of the bridge to the other. We have found that people are prepared to work hard to lose weight (or to keep it off). But people are not necessarily prepared to "work right." They know how to follow a diet regimen or an exercise regimen (and it would be fine to do either or both while you are working your way through this book). But, as we said at the start, this is not a diet book. No diet has a demonstrated track record of delivering *lasting* change—and it is actually not a criticism of any diet to say so.

A diet is a perfect example of a "technical fix." It goes directly at changing the behavior alone, and not the underlying challenge. To illustrate: Dr. Ronald Heifetz distinguishes between "technical" and "adaptive" challenges. The first can be met by new information, and changes to our behavioral routines or skill-sets alone. Adaptive challenges are different. They often require technical inputs as part of the solution (we need the information that teaches us what a "proper portion" is; we need some healthy, sensible diet that will spell out a new behavioral routine), but technical inputs alone will not enable us to meet any adaptive challenge because at their core, adaptive challenges require changes not just in our skill-sets but in our *mind-sets*. They require not just information but *transformation.*

For a lucky and tiny minority of us, losing weight and keeping it off may be a technical challenge. These are the people who decide to change the way they eat, lose the weight once, and never regain it. (Don't you love those people?) For the other 99% of us, losing weight is an adaptive challenge. **We will have to get the mind right to get the weight right**. Heifetz says our most common error is to try to meet adaptive challenges through technical means. For 99% of us, expecting dieting alone to get us to our goal is a form of that most common error.

We also predict that it will be hard for many of you to remember to keep your focus on changing your mind, and you will slip into focusing on your behavior. So we are going to remind you, again and again, in this book to refocus your attention on your mind. We may start to sound like a broken record, one that we hope will start to play in your own ear even when we stop reminding you.

The bridge we will help you build in the pages ahead will ensure that you address your adaptive challenge *with adaptive means*. That is what the immunity-to-change approach is meant to do. And the cynical publisher we quoted right at the beginning of this book is wrong: this approach is really not so hard once you understand what you are trying to do, and what to expect.

Before You Read On

We know we just ended with uplifting introductory remarks. But if we were betting folks, we'd wager that most of you will approach this book in similar ways to how you've previously tried to lose weight or become healthier—by using a "Diet Model." In this scenario, you've got the book in front of you and you are excited about the promise of *this* finally being the answer. You'll want to speed read through it so that you can find the gold nuggets and start following them immediately! And you hope to see the changes immediately! OK, maybe that's an exaggeration, but you get our point: to experience the benefits of this different approach to change, you need to take a different approach to it! We know, from experience, that the same work you are currently doing preventing your change can be turned to furthering it. Nothing extra is required. But it does take a proper stance.

Here's the approach we advise (and just in case you are worried, this is the most directive we will get).

- **Get prepared to write:** We have some tools for your use. Download the "Map Template" and "Change Journal" from http://www.mindsatwork.com before you start reading. You can also find a printed copy of these materials in the back of this book. Depending on your preference, you'll be writing your responses by hand or typing them into these materials.

- **Do the exercises!** This is your opportunity to apply the ideas to your personal situation, your own mind, your own behavior. Applying the ideas is key to your success with this approach. The ideas unto themselves—as novel and cool as they are—will not help you "work right."

- **Pace of reading:** It's fine to read and respond to Part One all in one week (that's the part of the book where we will coach you through creating your personal immunity-to-change (ITC) map. You might even want to read it more quickly. The threshold to cross before you move to Part Two is that you feel you have a powerful ITC map and it intrigues you. Once you get to the chapter "Practicing Self-Observation" in Part Two, it's best to read and work through only one chapter each week. It bears repeating: go slow so that you can go far. And deep. And without reverting to status quo.

It is true we are not going to move immediately toward changing your behavior or losing any weight in the first week. That is the appealing seduction of the technical approach. We are not going to put you on a path where you make linear incremental progress toward a goal of losing weight. We are first going to put you on a path where you make steady progress toward better understanding your own mind, and getting it right, so that you lose weight not temporarily but permanently; so that you change not just your weight but your whole relationship to food and eating. If you find yourself feeling impatient about the pace of things in the pages ahead, it is worth reminding yourself that you are embarking on a different course. If you envisioned taking a train from point to point it may feel like a waste of time that you are just sitting at the gate while the vehicle is being de-iced. The engine isn't running and it doesn't seem like you are getting anywhere. But when you finally get lift-off and you see you are not traveling by train at all, you will be glad you spent time de-icing the wings. You will be soaring at a different altitude, one that not only enables you to lose weight or keep it off, but one that reduces your suffering, one that brings you a new freedom.

PART ONE

Making Your Map

Well, we have kept you in suspense for long enough, and as promised we are now going to coach you to create your personal immunity-to-change (ITC) map. If you have been intrigued by the success stories that describe what others learned about themselves and the ways that they were undermining their own improvement goal, you may already be anticipating the way it will feel to discover something equally important about yourself. It's worth remembering: making these discoveries was *the* critical first step toward accomplishing their goals. It will be yours too!

We'll offer lots of examples of how other people – who were also trying to finally lose weight for good – came to their own answers. We'll suggest lots of things you can do that will help you arrive at the best answers for yourself.

Ready to get started? Let's go!

1

Naming Your Goals and Examining Your Behavior

How am I different after doing Immunity to Change? There are some things I avoid eating, like chocolate. I drink much less alcohol. I have become much more moderate in my eating, especially in the evening. In terms of quantity, I eat less, but I appreciate what I eat much more.

There are things I don't eat anymore because I don't desire them. I learned how to pay attention to what satisfies my appetite and my desires. I will absolutely maintain my weight because I changed my mind about eating.

—Claudia

In this chapter, we will give you an overview of the map-making process and then start guiding you step-by-step, showing you how to look more deeply into yourself for a very new understanding of why it is so difficult to lose weight and keep it off. The good news: making your ITC map is actually a simple and straightforward way to develop these powerful insights. You only need to be able to answer these five basic questions:

1. What are you committed to getting better at? This is your goal, the commitment you have that provides the motivation for you to be reading this book.
2. What are you doing (or not doing) that undermines your goal?
3. If you imagine even trying to do the opposite of those behaviors you just listed, what fears or worries arise for you?
4. Since you probably don't want to feel those fears or worries (let alone have them happen!) what

self-protective "hidden commitment" stands behind each of your fears and worries? (Don't expect to know the answer to this one right now.)

5. Finally, when you examine all that you have uncovered, what does that suggest about your assumptions – beliefs you hold about yourself and how things are – that connect to and support the answers you have to Questions 2-4? (We'll give you extra help with this one, too.)

In our experience, most people actually need a little help in coming to good answers to these questions. Maybe it is not even clear to you yet what we are asking with the last two. So here are some important suggestions to help you get started. We have found they make a lot of difference for many people.

Find a Good Partner

It's hard to think deeply about ourselves. It's usually very uncomfortable to look at our fears and expose hidden motivations. One of our clients once said that mapping her immunity to change was like realizing she had been walking around with her skirt tucked into the back of her underwear with her rear end hanging out for everyone to see. Nobody wants to feel that way! But when she said those words out loud, she laughed. And her coach laughed. They laughed because although the process can evoke feelings of vulnerability, that vulnerability also connected them in a shared sense of humanity.

What we reveal in our maps is almost never something completely unique to the mapmaker. That feeling of exposing a difficult, even embarrassing, part of ourselves is a feeling everyone has had. We all have big fears, and we all work hard to protect ourselves from shame, humiliation, and crisis. And it turns out that we do that in some very similar ways. We are not trying to suggest that we all have the same immunities, but over and over we have seen that when one person creates an honest and probing immunity-to-change map for herself, it speaks to something within all of us. Or, as Carl Rogers has said, "what is most personal is most universal." Above all else, the purpose of these explorations is not to leave us feeling uncomfortable, but to put us in a new position to realize goals that have long proved elusive.

A good partner in this process can help you get to your own truths. You can provide each other with emotional support. You can ask each other good questions. You can meet each other with curiosity and openness and compassion. You can give each other the space to give specific words to your intuitions, making them clearer and explicit. You can provide each other with accountability. Your partner should be someone you trust and are comfortable with, and is maybe even someone who also has a goal he or she has long tried to accomplish with little or only temporary success.

Let the Questions Marinate

Even with a partner it can still be hard to think deeply about ourselves. Insights are not like well-trained dogs – they don't just show up promptly whenever we call for them. You probably won't get full-blown and powerful answers the first time you read the questions or even the first time you sit down to focus on them. We have found that good answers often come when we least expect them. They come when we are mowing the lawn, lying awake in bed, taking a shower, or even when we are walking that well-trained dog. But that doesn't mean we should just ignore or distract ourselves from the questions. Instead, we recommend that you keep them somewhere close to the front of your mind — calling them up when you have a moment or two, turning them around in your head, maybe making notes on the thoughts that come up, and then letting them rest a bit.

So, you might make a first draft of your map and let that marinate. You might focus your thinking on one particular question if your answer doesn't feel full and rich and honest and true. Or you might try several strategies that allow you to reflect on some part of your map — talking with a few different people, for example. Or picking some particular times and places throughout your day when you want to raise these questions into your awareness. In those ways, you can develop a new and deeper awareness of yourself that leads to more powerful answers in your map.

Use the Provided Map Template to Record Your Answers

The picture you will create is a simple way to get at something quite complex – how you are unknowingly keeping yourself from reaching your improvement goal.

Think of the map as creating your own X-ray. X-rays are kind of amazing. They allow us to see through clothing, skin, and some tissues to our denser tissues and bones. They allow us to see clearly what we can't usually see at all – and so they help doctors to make a good diagnosis if we have a problem like a broken bone or an infection in our lungs. Our questions are designed to help you develop the X-ray vision that will allow you to see the complex workings underneath the surface of your goals, to see things about yourself that are usually deeply hidden. It is pretty common for people to be quite surprised by what shows up in their maps – beliefs and commitments and fears they often had no idea of before.

Column 1: Your Improvement Goal

Because you are reading a book about weight loss, we assume that your goals are focused in that area and perhaps more generally around enhancing your health and wellness. You may hope to lose 25 pounds (or 10 kilos), gain a new vitality and energy in your life, stop the endless cycle of dieting and then regaining, make exercise a regular part of your routine, or truly believe that you can achieve your goals. In order to do any of these things, you are going to have to get better at something:

- get better at planning your meals
- get better at eating slowly and stopping when you're full
- get better at maintaining a positive mindset
- get better at keeping a weekly exercise routine

Of course, there are many other possible examples we could list. But your personal map starts with how you would answer this question:

Question 1: What is the most important thing you need to get better at so as to achieve your own health and wellness goals?

This is your improvement goal. What do you want to get better at? Maybe you've read or heard weight loss advice that you know you should follow but can't? Maybe you have joined a weight loss program such as Weight Watchers or are following The South Beach Diet plan and are aware of the ways you are not faithfully adhering to their guidelines? Maybe your doctor has made specific recommendations like increasing your exercise that you haven't been able to follow? Listen carefully to your inner voice, as well, because you are making a commitment to yourself. What feels most motivating for you to get better at? What do you long to be able to do that would allow you to reach your goals? If you are barraged by advice from all sides, telling you what you need to get better at, what ultimately matters most to you?

We suggest that you write several possible improvement goals to start. We'll give you a few guidelines to then select the one that will work best for discovering your immunity.

Your improvement goal helps you to orient your X-ray, so it's important to select the right area to position the camera or else the picture you take won't end up being very useful to you. Now that you have a few possible improvement goals to choose from, let's help you choose one. The best improvement goal for this exercise should meet the following criteria:

- It should be about ***getting better at*** something, not a result or an outcome. "Losing 20 pounds" is not an improvement goal; it is a result or an outcome. "Getting better at eating proper portions" is an improvement goal (that could lead to losing 20 pounds).
- It should feel ***quite important to you***, so that you imagine its realization—if you can achieve it—as personally very valuable, desirable, or powerful.
- It should be something you have ***not yet accomplished***, meaning that there is plenty of room for improvement and future growth.
- It should be clear how getting better at this improvement goal means ***that YOU (not someone else) must make some changes to the way you live, think, and act.***

Review your various improvement goals and choose one that meets all of these criteria. Having a hard time deciding? Talk to your partner, if you are working with one. Or read the upcoming examples of Miriam, Ron and Maya and see if that helps. When you are ready, write your improvement goal in the first column of your map template. (If you haven't yet downloaded the template from our website, please do so now. Or use the map template in the Change Journal in the back of this book).

Improvement Goals: Miriam, Ron and Maya

Let us introduce you to Miriam, one of our ITC clients. Coming up with improvement goals seemed pretty easy to her. She had tried just about every major diet approach and knew quite a lot about all the things she was supposed to be doing. But after making a long list of goals, she felt overwhelmed and confused. Should she be trying to eat more complex carbs or no carbs at all? Should she try to boost her metabolism by going to the gym more often for high intensity workouts or by adding in low-intensity exercise like walking? More intermittent fasting or more small meals per day? Finally, she drew a big X through the entire list and asked herself, "If I throw all that out and just start with my own basic desires, what do I most want to get better at?" Here is her answer:

Miriam

COLUMN 1	COLUMN 2	COLUMN 3	COLUMN 4
My Improvement Goal			
• I'm committed to getting better at creating and following new lifelong food habits – no fad diets, no drastic approaches that I can't keep up.			

Another client, Ron, hadn't been working to lose weight for very long, but he was well aware of what he needed to improve. He could stick to healthy eating and exercise habits when he was alone and following a predictable routine. But whenever he was eating with others, he felt like he lost control of his ability to make his own choices. He would eat what others ate, what he felt like people wanted him to eat, or what others gave him to eat.

Ron

COLUMN 1	COLUMN 2	COLUMN 3	COLUMN 4
My Improvement Goal			
• I'm committed to getting better at eating healthier when I'm around other people – at the bar, at parties, at meetings where there is food.			

Maya also had a hard time coming up with the right improvement goal for her. She knew what she wanted — to lose 35 pounds before her high school reunion— but she didn't feel like she knew exactly what she needed to get better at to reach that goal. She hated joining groups, and she didn't really like the idea of talking to her doctor. Some people were hard to talk to. But she did have a friend at work, and they were often quite open with each other about their failed attempts to lose weight. She decided she would bring up the issue with Abigail and see if that would help her get some ideas about her own improvement goal. Maybe Abigail would want to do this immunity work together.

Talking to Abigail did help Maya name her improvement goal. It wasn't so much what Abigail said, but just listening to herself describe how and when she did most of her unhealthy eating made Maya realize what the problem was... and what she needed to get better at if she wanted to lose weight.

Maya

COLUMN 1	COLUMN 2	COLUMN 3	COLUMN 4
My Improvement Goal			
• I'm committed to making better food choices and being more active.			

Come On, Try It! You're reading on without having entered your goal, aren't you? If you really want this book to work for you, then the last thing you should do is "read" it, like you would a story. We love stories too, but that's not why we made this book. We made it for one reason – to bring you the new approach to change we have seen make spectacular differences in people's lives.

Column 2: What You Are Doing and Not Doing

Your next step requires brutal honesty. You need to develop a list of all the ***things you do*** that work against your improvement goal, as well as the ways you are working against that goal by ***what you are not doing***. In other words, we are asking you to tell on yourself — to be willing to fess up to your own "bad behaviors." Rest assured, we all have cheated on our diets. We all have intended to go to the gym but then decided to take a nap instead. We all have told ourselves we will resist the amazing desserts at our favorite restaurant. But then we eat them anyway. In other words, your list is going to be a picture of you working against your improvement goal. What are the things you are doing and not doing instead?

Question 2: What are you doing that undermines your goal? And similarly, what do you not do that undermines your goal?

Here are two criteria for this column:

- Be sure that the entries you list are ***behaviors***, and the more concrete you can be, the better. For example, rather than writing "I don't like diets," write something like, "I don't ever stick to a diet" or "I cheat," both of which are behaviors. Or instead of writing "I get bored eating only healthy foods," write something like, "I eat the same boring foods every day." If you find yourself naming something that is more like a feeling, a state of mind, or an attitude, just ask yourself, "What do I do (or what don't I do) that leads to these feelings or attitudes? What do I *do* (or not do) as a result of these feelings or attitudes?"

- Each item is **something that works *against*** your improvement goal. Our bet is that you are doing lots of things in order to move towards your improvement goal, but here we are asking you just the opposite! You'll see when we move to the next step in developing your X-ray how helpful it is to name what you do and don't do that *moves you away from your goal.*

The more behaviors you can list, the better your chances are of coming to powerful insights later in the process. So give yourself plenty of time to think back to all the times when you have sabotaged your intentions to lose weight, or to keep it off once you did lose it. What are the specific things you do and don't do?

Enter all of your answers to this question in the second column of your map template.

Finished with your list? When you have, review it carefully to make sure it is thorough, that all the entries are concrete behaviors, and that all of the *behaviors* listed work *against* your improvement goal.

It's useful to know that the two most common ways people go off track in this column are that they enter either explanations for why they are undermining their goals or what they plan to do differently. If you found either of these in your list, change them now and know that you are in good company! It is tempting to immediately start vowing and plotting to make things different. People usually feel guilty or embarrassed by their doing/not doing list and want to eradicate their list by being stricter with themselves, punishing themselves for their "bad behaviors," or willing themselves to be more disciplined. We think we need Jillian Michaels ("America's toughest trainer") to come and yell at us so that we'll finally get off our butts and go to the gym. Most of us also want to justify our missteps — to look to circumstances beyond our control, or the ways that other people make things hard for us. If only our mothers had taught us to eat better! If only our spouse would join our exercise routine! We want you to catch these impulses to reach for rationalizations or start making plans to change. You're going to see that our approach is very different. Again, all that should be in your second column are the specific things you do and don't do that work against your improvement goal. No judgments, no explanations, no promises to yourself or future plans!

Doing and Not Doing: Miriam, Ron and Maya

Miriam's long history of failed dieting gave her plenty of ideas for how to answer this question. At first she began to list some obvious behaviors. "I eat too much sugar and fat. I eat big portions. I eat too many snacks." Of course these behaviors sabotaged her goal. But as her list got longer, she began to think not just about what and how and when she ate, but about other things she did that undermined her goal of developing health lifelong eating habits. She summarized the first part of her list into one behavior: "I don't keep up healthy eating habits (eat too much fat & sugar; eat big portions; eat snacks.)" Then she started adding other behaviors – ways of thinking or talking to herself that were also undermining her goal. "I set unrealistic goals (e.g., lose 5 pounds in one week). If I have one slip-up, I use that as an excuse to give up – and then I gorge myself. I criticize myself really harshly whenever I make a dieting mistake. I constantly compare myself to thin people who all seem better than me and then I eat to make myself feel better." When she got to the end of her list, she realized that all her entries were food related. What about exercise? "Well, I hate exercise," she told herself. "I hate the gym. I hate putting on workout clothes and seeing how terrible I look." She started to add these words to her list but then realized they weren't actually *behaviors*. She decided to change her entry simply to, "I don't exercise" and added that to the end of her list.

Miriam

COLUMN 1	COLUMN 2	COLUMN 3	COLUMN 4
My Improvement Goal	"Doing and Not Doing"		
• I'm committed to getting better at creating and following new lifelong food habits – no fad diets, no drastic approaches that I can't keep up.	• I don't keep up healthy eating habits (eat too much fat & sugar; eat big portions; eat snacks). • I set unrealistic goals (e.g., lose 5 pounds in one week). • If I have one slip-up, I use that as an excuse to give up – and then I gorge myself. • I criticize myself really harshly whenever I make a dieting mistake. • I constantly compare myself to thin people who all seem better than me, and then I eat to make myself feel better. • I don't exercise.		

Ron didn't have to think long to come up with his first behavior that worked against his weight loss improvement goal — "I eat what my friends eat." Immediately, he came to his own defense. "I eat really well when I'm just doing my normal things – buying my regular lunch at work or eating my meals at home. I used to have second helpings a lot, but I've even cut back on them. And I'm probably working out more now than I did for years." It was tempting to add these good behaviors, ones that he was quite proud of, to his list. But when he started to write, he saw that they weren't the kinds of things he was supposed to be listing. "Just things that undermine my goal," he reminded himself. That didn't seem quite fair – he felt he should get some credit for the ways he was actually working hard to eat better. But after a brief struggle with himself, he brought himself back again to his first entry, "I eat what my friends eat. And what else?" he asked. He began to add other behaviors —some things he was doing and some things he was not doing (but felt he should be doing) — to his list.

Ron

COLUMN 1	COLUMN 2	COLUMN 3	COLUMN 4
My Improvement Goal	"Doing and Not Doing"		
• I'm committed to getting better at eating healthier when I'm around other people – at the bar, at parties, at meetings where there is food.	• I eat what my friends eat. • I eat when I am having fun. • I drink too much beer, and then I eat even more. • I don't tell other people I'm trying to lose weight. • When I am talking to people, I don't think about what I am eating. I just keep putting the food in my mouth. • I eat what is on my plate, even if I'm not hungry anymore.		

Maya and Abigail began to talk about their answers to the second question. Abigail was a good listener, and Maya felt like she could think more clearly when she was talking to someone. Also, Abigail didn't try to interrupt Maya and offer her own ideas or advice, something Maya couldn't stand. That's why she never talked about her weight with doctors or nutritionists. That's why she would never join a weight loss program, where people might tell you all the things you needed to do differently. In fact, Maya enjoyed naming some of her behaviors that worked against her improvement goal – Abigail provided lots of sympathy, and the two women laughed at all the "forbidden behaviors" they liked to indulge in.

Maya

COLUMN 1	COLUMN 2	COLUMN 3	COLUMN 4
My Improvement Goal	"Doing and Not Doing"		
• I'm committed to making better food choices and being more active.	• I buy healthy stuff, but I always keep unhealthy stuff around too. • If I'm out, I'll make an excuse to stop at a convenience store for junk food. • I don't join a gym because I know I won't go. • I keep junk food in my desk at work, and I'll eat that instead of going to get something better. • I watch too much TV. • I drink soda instead of water.		

As you can see, each of our mapmakers persisted until they found at least six behaviors to list in Column 2. We hope your own list is equally thorough and revealing.

If you are like most people, at this point in the exercise you may want to immediately try to go after your "bad" behaviors, imagining that through stronger will, greater self-discipline, or some kind of overall character improvement you'll be able to change them. We want to remind you not to fall for such temptations! This advice is hard for many of us to believe because we have learned to link personal health habits with personal character. We associate obesity with laziness, sloppiness, and greed. We therefore assume that the "cure" for obesity is simply to redouble our efforts – to work harder, to exercise self-control, grit and determination, to practice virtue. As the Nike marketers would say, "Just Do It." In fact, you may find that the "work harder" message resonates with you because it provides you with motivation. It speaks powerfully to your very sincere desires to lose weight, to keep weight off, to change your relationship to food and exercise.

You may also have found yourself mentally solving the weight loss problems that Miriam, Ron, and Maya faced, as you imagined the good advice that somebody could give them. Maybe you were thinking Ron should just get a stronger backbone and stand up to his friends, so that they don't influence his choices? Or if he can't do that, then he should stop going out with his friends, so as to remove the temptation to eat and drink. Or, if that doesn't work, maybe he just needs to get "better" friends who are more supportive of his goals. Problem solved? Not likely.

We aren't suggesting that there is anything necessarily wrong with that advice. It could very well be the case that if Ron stopped hanging out with the guys so much, he might actually eat better and lose weight. For some people, taking this type of straightforward advice and acting on it will be all they need to reach their goals. For some people, losing weight is really as simple as deciding to cut calories and exercise more, making these changes a permanent part of their lifestyle. If that works for you, then you should certainly apply that advice. And you don't need this book.

But let's be honest. You're not one of these people. And you know what? Very, very few people are. You've already tried to change by taking advice. You've already tried "willpower." It may even have worked for a while, right? As we all know, even the simplest advice isn't so simple. Millions of us try to exercise more and eat more healthfully, and we may even succeed briefly. And then we don't. And like you, Ron has promised himself over and over to cut out all those behaviors that undermine his goals. And sometimes he succeeds. And then he doesn't. And for a very good reason...

Because there are a few commitments he holds — actually, commitments that "hold him" since Ron doesn't even know he has them — that have *everything* to do with why he doesn't lose weight. This is the very key to how Ida Rose and Tony came to the realizations you read about at the beginning of this book. Do you remember Ida Rose's? The commitment that "had her" was to staying overweight, to not attracting romantic attention, to not possibly being an object of desire in some man's mind. Tony's commitment was to not hurting his loving aunts, and to him not being hurt by their comments when he refused their lovingly prepared foods. Uncovering this "hidden commitment" is the key to how *you* are going to be able to make changes – lasting changes – you were never able to make before. And, as you will see in the next chapter, it has nothing at all to do with you increasing your willpower. (Right now, you are probably doubting you have hidden commitments, or trying to figure out what yours are. Don't bother. You can't directly "think your way" to your hidden commitments. That's why we say they are hidden.)

2

Making The Invisible Visible: Behold! Your Immunity To Change

For me, the food situation was a symptom of the other things that were going on inside me. I was in fear that something external would make me unloveable, that having less (being thin) would mean being unhappy. It wasn't until the map that I was systematically able to unlock things. Other approaches tell us we have this particular hidden belief or that obstacle. But ITC gave me a way to find mine and really own it.

After I lost all the weight, things changed. I don't keep a food diary. I don't count calories. I am able to listen to my body better because I can turn down the other noise. I focus less on the number on the scale and more about the way my clothes fit. Aesthetically, I like how my body looks now. I like how I am getting stronger, how I can achieve more athletically and meet my strength goals.

— Joe

Questions 3 to 5 are designed to help you identify and explore the fears, worries, and hidden commitments that may be undermining your progress. Pushing yourself to answer them honestly, completely, and courageously will help you uncover the ways you are unknowingly motivated by other forces and desires and fears – ones that act in direct opposition to your desire to "Just Do It." Your careful and thoughtful answers will lead you to the kinds of powerful and often unexpected insights we have been promising. Let's move on to Column 3 of your immunity map.

Naming Your Fears and Worries

Column 3 gives you a chance to imagine behaviors that are the opposite of what you are currently doing and not doing. The exercise then asks you to stand back and see how these new behaviors would make you feel. It's a safe "feeling experiment" that can yield profound results.

Question 3. If you imagine yourself doing (or even just *trying* to do) the opposite of the things you just listed in Column 2 of your ITC map, are there any fears or worries that arise for you?

Look at each of the behaviors you listed in Column 2. One by one, imagine yourself in the act of doing the opposite of what you listed. As you imagine what it would be like to do the exact opposite, or even to try to, what worries or fears come up for you?

Since this is the hardest and most important part of developing your X-ray, let's look at an example of what a powerful answer is to this question. Let's look at how Miriam approached it. Among her other behaviors she wrote in her "doing and not doing" list, Miriam said, "I constantly compare myself to thin people who all seem better than me, and then I eat to make myself feel better." As Miriam looked at that behavior, she asked herself, "What if I weren't constantly making these comparisons? Actually, what if I ***completely stopped*** comparing myself to thin people?" At first, this idea sounded great. Miriam imagined that stopping these comparisons would allow her to stop evaluating herself all the time, to stop always finding fault with the way that she was. As she thought about that possibility, Miriam could more clearly see that she *did* have some fear about what it would be like to do that.

"Well," she said, "that would be like letting myself off the hook in a way. That would be like thinking I was great, that I didn't need fixing. Like I was blind to all my faults. So what is my fear or worry...?" Her voice trailed off as she searched for the right way to explain what she meant. "I guess I'm afraid that I'd think I'm better than I am. I'm afraid I'd be happy with myself." As she said these words aloud, Miriam's face registered both shock and confusion. "That's crazy! I'm afraid of being happy?!" But she knew she was onto something, so she kept searching for how it was that this could be true. "I'm afraid I would *think* I'm OK, *think* things are great, but they really wouldn't be. Then when I found out that I'm really a mess, and things are terrible, that would be even more awful because I would have stupidly thought I was fine." Miriam's eyes flashed with anger and pain. Suddenly, all the energy seemed to drain from her body. "Yeah..." her voice trailed off to a whisper. "That's it. I'm afraid of being happy because the worst thing to me is being a fool, having other people see what's wrong with me, *and me not seeing it!*" Looking up to her coach, she laughed dryly. "Being messed up isn't nearly as humiliating to me as feeling I'm OK when others can see I'm not."

As you can see from this example, we've reached a crucial moment in the process. At this point, many people begin to feel very uncomfortable. They may begin to sweat, to feel tightness in their chest, or a touch of nausea. They may experience quite powerful and unpleasant emotions – like disgust, or shame, or dread. While all of these experiences are indeed unpleasant, we are telling you about them because they are just the kinds of reactions it is perfectly fine for you to have. You may not feel exactly like this, but we are hoping you'll feel something similarly uncomfortable, and we think that is actually a positive sign that you are coming to something powerful about yourself. So if you do not feel like you've reached a crucial point and have not come to something powerful for yourself, slow down and do some more thinking. We have some suggestions to help you do that.

Go for the gut. Typically, we spend a lot of energy trying to keep our fears at bay, trying to convince ourselves that we actually do not have fears but are instead only strong, capable, logical, calm, poised. If that's all you let yourself feel, you are not going to have a powerful map. So we invite you to reach down deep inside and try to come up with something at least a little bit scary that you can feel in your gut. When you do, it doesn't mean you are any less strong, capable, logical, calm or poised. It just means you are taking a closer look at the fears or anxieties you may be managing so well when you are strong, capable, logical, calm or poised.

Sometimes you can get to a deeper place by really **slowing down your reactions** and pushing yourself to imagine what is actually the *opposite* of (not just different from) your second column behaviors. To illustrate, let us tell you a bit about Ricardo, whose goal was to get in better shape by exercising more often. Ricardo was trying to come up with his fear by asking himself, "If I did go the gym regularly, *every day* even" (the opposite of one of his behaviors in Column 2), "what would I fear?" He shrugged and replied, "Nothing. It would be annoying, I guess. Inconvenient." That's all he could imagine. "That's why I don't do it more often. I just don't like doing it every day."

We tried slowing down his thinking, asking him to try to stay with the feeling of what it would be like to go every day, to be a regular at the gym, to be annoyed and feel inconvenienced for a bit and see if there was something even more uncomfortable bubbling up. Ricardo — looking up to the ceiling and concentrating hard — shrugged again. "It's just — you know, who has time for that? Who has time to do all the repetitions and work everything — you know arms, legs, back, stomach? I mean what kind of person enjoys that?" Now his tone grew scornful. "Those guys are all just stupid, really. They're just big bodies. So what? That's all they think about. Big bodies with small brains."

Ricardo's face and voice were growing animated, and he was gesturing more energetically with each sentence. He could see that his reaction to going to the gym regularly was stronger than he had initially thought. "Yeah, so what am I *afraid* of?" he wondered aloud. "I'm afraid of being some dumb jock on steroids? That big muscles will make my brain small? Yeah, maybe…" But there was more to it. "I mean, I have never liked guys like that. Those were the kind of guys who were very powerful when I was in school. They did whatever they wanted to and thought they were kings." Ricardo began speaking more quickly now. "Kings of everyone. I'm sure they are not now. But then, they could do what they wanted. And the best way for me was just to stay out of their way. I knew that was the only way to be left alone. I could be smart, and small, and not good at sports, and love reading and cooking only if I kept them from noticing me. Only if I made myself even smaller."

Ricardo was silent for a long time, nodding his head slowly as he thought. "You know what I am afraid of? I'll tell you. I am afraid that if I become a gym rat, I'll be like them. I'll like those kinds of guys. I'll feel like they were *right* all along – that they *did* have something that I didn't have. I'm afraid that I will be a dumb jock, that I'll like being a dumb jock, and that I'll feel like the other things that I have always been good at are less important. It's silly, isn't it?" Again, he was nodding slowly. "Yeah, but that's what it is."

What Ricardo had unearthed is what we call a "dreaded image," an idea of himself that he has been working pretty hard to avoid. If you are having trouble finding your fears, try slowing things down and really allowing your imagination to play out what it would feel like to do the opposite of what you listed in Column 2. If you are still having trouble, ask yourself, "As I imagine doing the opposite of each behavior in my second column, what is my 'dreaded image'?" Miriam's dreaded image, for example, is that she is "over-valuing" herself, not noticing flaws others can see, being clueless. A "dreaded image" is a way I would *least* like others to see me, or a way I would least like to see myself. What might you really hate for others to see in you (that they might see if you were doing the opposite of what is in your second column)? What might be a way you would least like to see yourself (if you were doing, or even trying to do, the opposite of something in your second column)?

Now it's your turn. Allow yourself to surface your fears or worries, ones that you can feel in your gut, and write these in the box in the top half of Column 3 in your map template. This is what we call your *worry box*.

Fears and Worries: Miriam, Ron and Maya

As we have already showed you, Miriam identified at least one fear: "believing that I'm OK when I'm really not" (and so being blind to her problems). That realization was important for her and led her to see how this same fear, and some closely related fears, was connected to her other behaviors. For example, Miriam realized, "If I was being realistic in my weight loss goals and was able to get quickly back on track when I slip up, I see that I'm actually afraid that I would succeed. I mean, it's like – what if I really do get this monkey off my back and get my life under control...? There's something actually terrifying about that. Because then what? I have no more excuses. I can't hide behind being fat. I'll have to really see myself and be seen by others for who I truly am. And that's terrifying," she admitted. "What if they reject me? What if I'm really me, and I'm still not good enough?" As she spoke those final words, Miriam's voice broke and she dropped her face into her hands. "You must think I'm crazy," she said finally. "I know I do."

Miriam

COLUMN 1	COLUMN 2	COLUMN 3	COLUMN 4
My Improvement Goal	"Doing and Not Doing"	Hidden Counter-Commitments	
• I'm committed to getting better at creating and following new lifelong food habits – no fad diets, no drastic approaches that I can't keep up.	• I don't keep up healthy eating habits (eat too much fat & sugar; eat big portions; eat snacks). • I set unrealistic goals (e.g., lose 5 pounds in one week). • If I have one slip-up, I use that as an excuse to give up – and then I gorge myself. • I criticize myself really harshly whenever I make a dieting mistake. • I constantly compare myself to thin people who all seem better than me, and then I eat to make myself feel better. • I don't exercise.	Worry box: I fear I will believe I am okay (when I'm clearly not!). I fear I will lose weight and have no excuses, nothing to hide behind. I will be exposed and rejected.	

Ron looked at the behaviors he listed and tried to imagine doing the opposite. "What if I let people know that I'm trying to eat healthy? What if I go out with friends and had just one or two beers and didn't have the nachos or a burger and fries?" He knew right away what worried him. "I know what they'd say," he explained, "they'd tease me for being on a diet, like I'm a girl. They'd joke around offering me a salad or asking if I thought their pants made their asses look big. You know, like I was a girl. They'd just keep it up and keep it up until I either ate the nachos or got so mad I shoved them down their throats." Ron rolled his head to loosen the muscles in his neck and exhaled sharply. "Even if they don't make fun of me, I will just feel weird, like I'm not really hanging out with guys if I'm not also enjoying the cheese-steaks. The food is actually a big part of our experiences, especially at sports events. It's just what we do together. It's how we have fun."

Ron

COLUMN 1	COLUMN 2	COLUMN 3	COLUMN 4
My Improvement Goal	"Doing and Not Doing"	Hidden Counter-Commitments	
• I'm committed to getting better at eating healthier when I'm around other people – at the bar, at parties, at meetings where there is food.	• I eat what my friends eat. • I eat when I am having fun. • I drink too much beer, and then I eat even more. • I don't tell other people I'm trying to lose weight. • When I am talking to people, I don't think about what I am eating. I just keep putting the food in my mouth. • I eat what is on my plate, even if I'm not hungry anymore.	Worry box: I worry that my friends will taunt me about being like a girl. I worry that I'll have to stop hanging out with them completely. I worry that I won't feel like I am part of the group, no matter what they do.	

Maya and Abigail decided to take a walk during their lunch hour to talk about their fears. Since they had similar second column behaviors, they figured their fears might be the same too. But as Maya listened to Abigail talk, she knew that their fears were different. The more she listened, the clearer she got about what her own fears were. As Abigail talked about fearing losing the joys and pleasures of her life (by depriving herself of the foods and bad habits she enjoyed and felt she deserved), Maya bit her tongue to stop from interrupting. Finally, Abigail paused and said, "Is that what you came up with too?" Maya was quick to jump in with an emphatic, "No way!" When Abigail recoiled, Maya realized she probably should have softened her response.

"I mean, I get what you're saying, Abigail." She added hastily, "I love that stuff too, right? But here's the real thing for me. Every time I try to go on a diet, I feel like someone is watching over my shoulder and scolding me whenever I even think about food. It just makes it worse, actually. I feel like I'm always hungry and always mad that I can't have what I really want." Suddenly she saw there *was* a connection between her fears and Abigail's. "Maybe that is like what you said — that I feel like I should eat whatever I want, and do whatever I want. *That's* what I deserve. I deserve to make my own choices!" So their fears weren't exactly the same, but they both felt they deserved something they couldn't have if they dieted.

Hearing Abigail talk had helped Maya see that about herself. She went on, "Then my *fear*, I guess, is that somebody else thinks I can't make my own choices... My fear is following somebody's rules – not mine – for how to live *my* life. I would feel like someone is trapping me or holding me back from something." Maya knew this was exactly the fear she held. After all, wasn't she always fighting with her husband whenever she felt like he was trying to tell her what to do? No matter how good his advice might be, Maya always initially rejected his ideas... because they were *his* ideas. It had long been a sore point between them. Yes, she was 100% sure that she had named her biggest fear.

Maya

COLUMN 1	COLUMN 2	COLUMN 3	COLUMN 4
My Improvement Goal	"Doing and Not Doing"	Hidden Counter-Commitments	
• I'm committed to making better food choices and being more active.	• I buy healthy stuff, but I always keep unhealthy stuff around too. • If I'm out, I'll make an excuse to stop at a convenience store for junk food. • I don't join a gym because I know I won't go. • I keep junk food in my desk at work, and I'll eat that instead of going to get something better. • I watch too much TV. • I drink soda instead of water.	Worry box: I fear spending my life having to follow someone else's rules. I fear being categorized as either a "good" girl or a "bad" girl, depending on what I eat.	

Uncovering Your Hidden Commitments

If your answers to Question 3 named fears that you could feel in your gut, this next question will be somewhat easier for you—but your next answers still need to evoke your sense of danger. If, despite your sincere efforts, your fears haven't quite reached the gut level, you may be able to do something about that here. You'll notice on your map that the worry box only covers the top part of Column 3 and that there is plenty of space below it for your answers to Question 4. That's because your answers to Questions 3 and 4 are closely connected. Identifying your fears and worries will help you discover something else—what we call a "hidden competing commitment."

It makes perfect sense that it is hard or uncomfortable for us to identify our fears and worries. Nobody wants to feel fear or worry. We don't generally enjoy experiencing ourselves as in danger or at risk in some way. We don't often seek out that kind of vulnerability. Instead, we usually try to protect ourselves from these feelings. We defend ourselves from what terrifies us. We make sure that not only are we *not* standing on the edge of our own personal abyss of anxiety and danger but that we are standing quite comfortably far, far away... far enough away so we don't even have to be consciously aware that the abyss is there.

From a psychological perspective, our hidden commitments are our mental strategies for standing far away from the abyss, our ways of keeping far away from the things we fear. We are not usually conscious of these commitments – to be conscious of them would mean we would also have the uncomfortable awareness of our fears. So they usually stay "hidden" from consciousness, all the while working hard to make sure the things we are afraid of do not happen.

Ricardo didn't go to the gym regularly not just because he feared that he'd become something he had always hated–a dumb jock who abuses power–and lose the familiar sense of himself as a smart, sensitive guy. He didn't go to the gym because he didn't even want *to feel* that fear, didn't want to have that uneasiness in the pit of his stomach day after day. Instead, Ricardo was effectively, actively, even *brilliantly* protecting himself from finding out that he could be the very thing he hated. He was protecting himself *even from the fear* that he would find out he could be the very thing he hated. The best way for Ricardo to protect himself was to stay away from the gym… to make sure that whatever else he did, he did not go there regularly. By *not* going to the gym regularly, he did not have to feel the unpleasant fear he associated with becoming a gym rat. In this way not going to the gym was actually effectively solving a problem for Ricardo. Not going to the gym beautifully kept his fears at bay. Unfortunately, not going to the gym also undermined his weight loss goals.

Now we can see why all the good advice in the world for someone like Ricardo–or Ron, or Miriam, or Maya, or the millions of us who are also trying unsuccessfully to lose weight or maintain a weight loss–doesn't work. We can see clearly how Ricardo can't just *will* himself to the gym because the more he goes, the more uncomfortable he will actually get. It is as if he is sitting behind the wheel of a car with his right foot on the gas and his left foot on the brake. His right foot is working on his improvement goal, the part of him that wants to lose weight by going to the gym more often. He steps on the gas, trying to speed up, to get more momentum going in the direction he'd like to be moving. He steps down even harder. The car engine is revving. The car is even shaking as it holds this increased force. But the car isn't actually going anywhere. Why?

The car isn't going anywhere because Ricardo's left foot won't let it move. The harder his right foot presses on the gas (by making plans and resolutions to go to the gym), the harder his left foot steps on the brake. The foot on the brake is working to make sure he does not become a gym rat, does not become the dumb jock who abuses power that some part of Ricardo is worried he could become. Until he looked deeper into his "bad behavior" of not going to the gym, Ricardo was not consciously aware of how powerful his fears were about how he might change were he to go to the gym regularly. He had no idea that there was this other part of himself (his left foot on the brake) working in complete opposition to his goals, competing with them. He had no sense whatsoever of how intelligent, reasonable, and faithful he was being to this hidden part of himself every time he did not go to the gym. This hidden part, this hidden, competing commitment, was protecting him from the doubts he had about his own identity and his own motivations. "I am committed to not finding out what I would be like if I had physical power, to not finding out that in my heart, I am just as mean and abusive as the dumb jocks I grew up with."

Ricardo

COLUMN 1	COLUMN 2	COLUMN 3	COLUMN 4
My Improvement Goal	"Doing and Not Doing"	Hidden Counter-Commitments	
• I'm committed to getting in better shape by losing a few pounds and exercising regularly.	• I join gyms but then I don't go. • I quit every gym I join. • I sign up for sessions with a personal trainer and then cancel them. • I schedule time in my day to go the gym during lunch but then I find an excuse so that I "can't go."	Worry box: I am afraid that if I become a dumb jock, the other things that I have always been good at will be less important. I am committed to not finding out what I would be like if I had physical power, to not recognizing that in my heart, I am just as mean and abusive as the dumb jocks I grew up with.	

If you look at the relationship between your Column 1 improvement goal and your Column 3 hidden commitments, you'll see two powerful forces working in opposition. Each force is generating lots of energy, with the net effect of keeping Ricardo in the exact same place — immune to change. In fact, there is a single "system" at work across the three columns. This is what we call an "immune system" because we believe the mind, like the body, has an immune system – an invisible, ceaseless dynamic that exists for one purpose: to keep us out of trouble, to protect us, even to save our lives.

It is important, therefore, to see that the picture that is about to emerge on your own map is not a picture of something *wrong* with you. An immune system is not an illness, disease, weakness, or problem that needs to be fixed or cured. An immune system is an intelligent, beautiful phenomenon that only wants to take care of you. However, our immune systems – physical or mental – can still get us in trouble, even when they are working on our behalf. When the immune system is in error, when it sees a danger that is not there, it will go to work "protecting" us from the very awareness we may need in order to thrive.

Like Ricardo, you now have a different way of understanding your obstructive second column behaviors. If you look at each of the fears you identified in your worry box, you'll see that they can be converted into "hidden competing commitments." These are "commitments" preventing the things you fear from occurring, and we aren't usually aware that we have them. As well, they are different from our improvement goals because they aren't something we hope to fulfill in the future. Without even knowing it, we are already fulfilling them right now! If your worry box holds something like, "I'm afraid if I don't eat whatever I want, I will lose all the pleasure in my life," then you might convert that into a commitment like, "I am committed to feeling the pleasure I get from eating." Or, "I am committed to not losing any of the pleasure I get from food." Or perhaps, "I am committed to not having to give food as the biggest (or only?) pleasure in my life." Try on different versions to see which one feels most powerful and most true for you. Then move on to the next fear you have listed and convert it into a hidden commitment too.

Question 4: Since you probably don't want to experience those fears or worries (let alone have them happen!) what self-protective hidden commitment stands behind each of your fears or worries?

Here are three guidelines to help you come to a good answer to this question:

- **Keep the fear, worry, or dread from the worry box when you convert it into a hidden commitment.** For example, "I fear others will think I'm not up to this job" should be converted to "I'm committed to others not thinking poorly of me" or "I'm committed to not being seen as incompetent" and **not** "I'm committed to others thinking well of me" or "I'm committed to being seen as competent." You may need to use a clunky double negative in order to preserve the danger you are protecting yourself from, and that's fine!

- **Hidden commitments are forms of self-protection.** They protect us from the dangers that may lurk in our fears. Miriam has a hidden commitment to not be clueless about her own deficiencies. That commitment protects her from a fear that, for her, is worse than others' disdain – namely the fear of being blindsided.

- **Hidden commitments should show how the behaviors you have listed in Column 2 make perfect sense!** Powerful hidden commitments mean that those "bad behaviors" are also simultaneously very, very "good behaviors," making sure that one foot stays firmly on the brake.

Now it's your turn. Take each one of your fears or worries and convert them into "hidden competing commitments." Write your answer in the bottom half of Column 3 in your map template (underneath where you wrote your worries and fears).

Once you have identified your own hidden commitments you should now see a whole picture across your three columns, a picture of your personal immunity to change. It should show you what your own left foot is doing, how it is stepping on the brake and keeping your right foot from moving the car forward. You should have arrived at something that intrigues you because it sheds new light on the struggles you have been having with your weight. That doesn't mean you will know yet how to solve this problem, how to end the struggling. That will come later. Einstein said that if he had one hour to save the world, he would spend 55 minutes defining the problem and only 5 minutes finding the solution. That is because we can't get to the right solution if we don't truly understand the problem. You will come to a solution, but only after you have gotten the problem right.

The problem is *not* that you can't change your behavior. The problem is not that you are weak-willed; you are very *strongly* taking good care of yourself. The problem is that the perfectly sensible unconscious effort to take care of yourself is producing the very behaviors guaranteed to keep you from accomplishing your goal!

Seeing the problem in this new way should make your sheet of paper now appear valuable, not just a bunch of words on a page, but a detailed map of your personal immunity to change. It should show you how you have one foot pressing the gas toward fulfilling your weight loss improvement goal, and one foot on the brake to fulfill your hidden competing commitment. If your map does not yet feel intriguing, what might help? Make sure the fear, worry, or dread from the worry box did not disappear when you converted it into a hidden commitment. That will mean that the "virus" or danger the immune system is protecting you from did not get named in your hidden commitments. Remember that clunky "double negatives" are fine; this isn't an English class!

When you look at your hidden commitments, you should be able to see how you have been protecting yourself. If not, spend some time thinking, "What is the danger lurking for me? In what way am I trying to protect myself?" Let these questions marinate. Talk to your partner.

Look to see if everything you identified as a hidden commitment also shows how the behaviors you listed in Column 2 now make perfect sense. You should be able to see why it hasn't (and won't) work to try to change those behaviors only through willpower or increased effort. The harder you step on the gas, the harder your other foot will step on the brakes. You will be spending more energy trying to go in opposite directions at the same time. If you can't see how your hidden commitments make your behaviors in Column 2 look perfectly reasonable, that's a sign that you've gotten off track somewhere. You may need to revise your hidden commitments or go back to your fears to see if you need to get clearer about them.

Take a look at the chart at the end of this chapter. It shows some of the most common hidden fears and competing commitments we have encountered with our clients, and perhaps one or more of these will help you to put your finger on your fears and competing commitments.
It may help to consider Miriam, Ron and Maya's experiences. That's where we are heading next.

Hidden Commitments: Miriam, Ron and Maya

Miriam hated having to write her fears into her immunity map. "I fear that I will believe I am OK (when I'm clearly not!). I fear that I will lose weight and have no excuses, nothing to hide behind. I will be exposed and rejected." Seeing them in print made her feel even more vulnerable and silly. But it wasn't hard for her to figure out what her hidden commitments were. They seemed to be suddenly staring her in the face, and she quickly named several that were all directly connected to her fears: "I am committed to not being clueless or blindsided about the ways I am screwed up. I am committed to not losing being fat as an excuse," Miriam explained. "As long as I am fat, that can be the reason why I am not happy." She continued, "I am committed to hiding behind my weight. As long as I am fat, I shouldn't really try to get what I want in life. I am committed to having no one see 'the real me.' I am committed to not letting anyone reject 'the real me.'" She looked up from her map, shaking her head, "I guess in some way, I want to be fat. I must be crazy."

Miriam

COLUMN 1	COLUMN 2	COLUMN 3	COLUMN 4
My Improvement Goal	"Doing and Not Doing"	Hidden Counter-Commitments	My Big Assumptions
• I'm committed to getting better at creating and following new lifelong food habits – no fad diets, no drastic approaches that I can't keep up.	• I don't keep up healthy eating habits (eat too much fat & sugar; eat big portions; eat snacks). • I set unrealistic goals (e.g., lose 5 pounds in one week). • If I have one slip-up, I use that as an excuse to give up – and then I gorge myself. • I criticize myself really harshly whenever I make a dieting mistake. • I constantly compare myself to thin people who all seem better than me, and then I eat to make myself feel better. • I don't exercise.	Worry box: I fear I will believe I am okay (when I'm clearly not!). I fear I will lose weight and have no excuses, nothing to hide behind. I will be exposed and rejected. • I am committed to not being clueless or blindsided about the ways I am screwed up. • I am committed to not losing being fat as an excuse. • I am committed to hiding behind my weight. • I am committed to not letting up on myself. • I am committed to not letting anyone reject 'the real me.'	

Ron struggled a bit to figure out how to convert his fears to commitments. He looked at his worries: "I worry that my friends will taunt me about being like a girl. I worry that I'll have to stop hanging out with them completely." So: "I'm committed to not being a girl? I'm committed to having friends?" He knew these didn't sound right, didn't really have a powerful impact on him. He thought for a long time, asking himself, "What am I protecting myself from? What would be the worst thing that could happen?" He turned these questions around and around in his head and kept coming back to the same idea. "I don't want my friends to think I'm weird. That's basically it. I don't want to be the weird guy." So how to write this as a commitment? "I guess," Ron said, shrugging his shoulders, "it's pretty simple. I just want to fit in and be one of the guys."

Saying these words out loud was not difficult or upsetting for Ron. As he said them, he knew with certainty that wanting to fit in was exactly what was behind the overeating and overdrinking he did each time he went out with his friends. In fact, he felt a little hopeless about how he was ever going to get healthy because he knew that he would never be able to accept being "the weird guy." "If that's what it takes to eat better, I'm in trouble," he groaned. "This is probably why all of America is overweight now. I mean, nobody wants to be the weird guy."

Ron

COLUMN 1	COLUMN 2	COLUMN 3	COLUMN 4
My Improvement Goal	"Doing and Not Doing"	Hidden Counter-Commitments	
• I'm committed to getting better at eating healthier when I'm around other people – at the bar, at parties, at meetings where there is food.	• I eat what my friends eat. • I eat when I am having fun. • I drink too much beer, and then I eat even more. • I don't tell other people I'm trying to lose weight. • When I am talking to people, I don't think about what I am eating. I just keep putting the food in my mouth. • I eat what is on my plate, even if I'm not hungry anymore.	Worry box: I worry that my friends will taunt me about being like a girl. I worry that I'll have to stop hanging out with them completely. I worry that I won't feel like I am part of the group, no matter what they do. • I am committed to fitting in with my friends, to not being one of the "weird guys." • I am committed to not being cast out from the group.	

Maya's first hidden commitment followed closely from her fears. "I fear spending my life following someone else's rules" quickly converted to "I am committed to breaking the rules." Then she tried a slightly different version: "I am committed to living without rules." Yes, that was even better. "What about your fear of being a good girl or bad girl?" asked Abigail. Maya thought about that for a moment. "It's the same – committed to living without rules." But she paused because she saw that this wasn't exactly right.

There was also something about doing what other people wanted her to do... and something else too. She started talking it through. "I just don't think I am good at diets because I feel so boxed in. Like everybody should eat the same thing, and it all tastes like boiled chicken, and I feel like I am supposed to like that. And I don't! And they are all idiots if they think people like that crap! I know what tastes good to me, and *I want to decide* when to eat and how much, and I don't want anybody weighing me or checking up on me or telling me what to make for lunch." Abigail nodded. "So you're committed to...?" "I'm committed to running my own life. I'm committed to... being in control. I'm committed to knowing I'm right." Maya laughed at that last one. "And believe me, I think I'm right about everything."

Abigail looked puzzled and then slowly said, "Maya, I don't get it. How does wanting to be in control and right keep you from eating better? If you want to be right, wouldn't you be eating right all the time?" Maya smiled. "You would think I would," she said. "But all those diets and doctors and weight-loss commercials just make me want to do the opposite of what they say. I don't want to listen to them. I don't want those idiots telling me what to do. So I do what I want because..." she groped for words, "because at least then I show them they're wrong... or something." Maya paused again. "I know – it makes no sense. It's not like I'm actually *thinking* about this when I do it. It just happens."

Maya

COLUMN 1	COLUMN 2	COLUMN 3	COLUMN 4
My Improvement Goal	"Doing and Not Doing"	Hidden Counter-Commitments	
• I'm committed to making better food choices and being more active.	• I buy healthy stuff, but I always keep unhealthy stuff around too. • If I'm out, I'll make an excuse to stop at a convenience store for junk food. • I don't join a gym because I know I won't go. • I keep junk food in my desk at work, and I'll eat that instead of going to get something better. • I watch too much TV. • I drink soda instead of water.	Worry box: I fear spending my life having to follow someone else's rules. I fear being categorized as either a "good" girl or a "bad" girl, depending on what I eat. • I am committed to running my own life, not following someone else's rules. • I'm committed to not giving up control. • I'm committed to not being the "bad" girl in the dieting world.	

At this point we hope that you feel you are approaching something that is both powerful and intriguing for you. People sometimes remark to us how mapping their immunity to change *quickly* gets them to a deep level of insight and awareness about how they are stuck. Others need a bit more time and help in order to get to something that feels meaningful. So at this point it is worth asking yourself, "On a scale of 1-5 (where "1" means "not powerful" or "not intriguing" and "5" means "very powerful" or "very intriguing"), how does this map feel for me?" If you answered "4" or "5," that's great, and you should feel free to move on to question 5 in the next chapter. If you answered "1," "2," or "3," we recommend that you get a little help to strengthen your entries. If the map doesn't "pop" for you, there is probably a problem in one or more columns. You'll find help at the end of the Chapter 3 in the section titled "Making Your Map More Powerful." Once your map feels more powerful, then turn to the beginning of Chapter 3.

Common Fears and Hidden Commitments

Type of Issue: Loss or Harm in My Relationships with Others

I fear...	I am also committed to...
• Losing others' acceptance, not fitting in • Losing others' approval, respect • Being rejected • Being criticized or judged • Letting others down, disappointing their expectations • Becoming exactly what others have expected me to be • Receiving unwanted attention or approval • Causing conflict or chaos • Putting myself first, looking or being selfish • Losing social power • Giving others the impression that I am judging them • Being rude or ungrateful	• Not being rejected by others, not being the outcast • Not being disapproved of by others, disrespected, not being rejected • Not allowing others to see who I really am • Not letting others down or disappointing them • Not becoming the person others expect me to be • Not receiving (unwanted) attention or approval • Not causing conflict or chaos • Not being or looking selfish, putting my own needs last • Not losing social power • Not having others think I am judging them • Not being seen as rude or ungrateful

Type of Issue: Control

I fear...	I am also committed to...
• Losing my free will • Losing control • Being vulnerable • Proving that I am weak, that I have no self-control, willpower, discipline • Living in chaos	• Not surrendering free will, choice • Not losing control • Not being vulnerable • Not finding out or proving to others that I am weak, have no self-control, willpower, or discipline • Not causing chaos or being overwhelmed by chaos

Type of Issue: Uncomfortable Emotions or Inner States

I fear...	I am also committed to...
• Feeling denied, deprived, bored, or burdened • Increased stress • Emotional pain, discomfort, insecurity • Loss of food as a way to feel better and self-soothe • Loss of joy, pleasure, self-reward, relaxation • That I will be too proud, positive, full of myself • That I will not be any happier	• Not feeling denied, deprived, bored, or burdened • Not feeling over-run with distress • Not having to feel emotional pain, discomfort, insecurity • Not losing food as a way to feel better, self-soothe • Not losing food as a way to experience joy, pleasure, self-reward, relaxation • Keeping myself small, not being too full of myself or seen as too full of myself • Not finding out I won't be any happier

Type of Issue: Identity

I fear...	I am also committed to...
• Not being the same person I have been • Feeling as though I don't exist • Becoming a completely different person • Having to sacrifice a part of myself (inner child, role as good wife, good mother)	• Not losing identity • Not feeling I don't exist, that I am insignificant or invisible • Not changing anything about myself, not becoming different

Type of Issue: Gender Expectations

I fear...	I am also committed to...
• That I will be fitting into, upholding, or benefiting harmful expectations for how I/we should look or act	• Not losing my stance as outsider, on the margins, social critic

Type of Issue: Results, Outcomes

I fear...	I am also committed to...
• That I will succeed • That I will fail • Letting myself down • Having others think I am a failure • That I will have no excuses	• Not finding out that I can succeed • Not running the risk of failure • Not finding out I am not as good as I think I am • Not looking like a failure • Not losing my excuses

Type of Issue: Scarce Resources

I fear...	I am also committed to...
• That I won't have enough time • That I will have to sacrifice something else	• Not feeling continuously short on time • Not reworking my schedule, my habits and routines, my lifestyle

Type of Issue: Physical

I fear...	I am also committed to...
• Injury • Illness • Weakness	• Not taking any physical risks, or making myself ill, vulnerable • Not seeing myself as weak, unhealthy, sedentary

3

UNCOVERING YOUR BIG ASSUMPTIONS

When Tomas tried to identify his hidden commitments, he imagined doing the opposite of what was in his second column. "What if I did not eat what my wife buys and prepares? I worry I would not be showing my appreciation for her efforts in caring for the family. She buys what she thinks I like and enjoy eating." He then identified his hidden commitment, "I'm committed to not disappointing my wife."

But Tomas had a nagging feeling that he had not yet gotten to the heart of the matter. Again, he thought about the fears and worries that would arise for him if he changed his eating habits. It took a lot of brooding and inner searching before he found the right words. "I worry I would feel deprived, like I don't have enough compensation for leading a stressful life. I worry I would feel like I do not have enough recognition or reward. I would not have enough pleasure in my life to make all my sacrifices worthwhile." Now he was getting to a deeper level of his immunity. "I am committed to not feeling deprived of pleasure and success. I am committed to not preventing myself from having the rewards and relaxation I deserve. I am committed to not sacrificing so much of myself without also having clear signs that I am a success." Now he understood the secret he had been keeping for himself.

If you've been able to dig deep enough, by now we hope you have come to an important realization: why it is that you haven't been able to lose weight and keep it off. You may be thinking, "OK, now what?" Well, now you know why all your previous diets have failed. You know why every time you lose weight, you gain it back. You know why the sure-fire weight loss approach that worked for your neighbor doesn't work for you. You know why simply working harder – or having more self-discipline or willpower — will not get you any closer to your goals. And we know, we know: all that probably doesn't make you feel one bit better! All we have shown you is exactly why you have this weight loss problem. For some of you, it may even feel we have made your problem seem worse. "I started off thinking I couldn't lose weight," complained Miriam with a weary laugh, "and now I am sure *everything* about me is a mess!"

There is a reason why we've spent all this time getting to a clearer picture of what the problem really is. That is because it is only when you can see more deeply into how it is — and why it is — you have been preventing yourself from losing weight or keeping it off that you enter a whole new space to begin changing. Only when you have an accurate "mental map" can you correctly see where the obstacles are so that you can chart the course ahead. So you have created a vividly clear, and perhaps painfully clear, personally powerful map of the problem. Now you can start working on creating your own personally powerful solution.

Your Big Assumptions

The most effective solution goes right to the heart of the matter – starting not with the behaviors that need to be changed, but with the core assumptions that hold your immune system in place, the "roots" of your behaviors. Assumptions are basically beliefs, ideas that we have about ourselves and about the world. But because we tend to take these beliefs as *truths*, as rules about how the world really is, we call them "Big Assumptions." (We will use that term and the shortcut, "BA," interchangeably for the rest of the book.)

Ricardo assumes, for example, that there is a dark, untrustworthy, power-hungry part of himself that would be unleashed if he went to the gym regularly. He believes that the more he goes to the gym, the more likely it is that this terrible part of himself would be fed and would take over. If you do not hold a similar assumption about yourself, you may think it is a little silly of Ricardo to believe such a thing. In fact, many of Ricardo's friends would be shocked to hear of his assumption. To them, Ricardo is a sweet, sensitive, smart person — the farthest they can think of from a mean, "dumb jock" who abuses his power.

But this assumption is very real to Ricardo. Part of him can actually see that it is silly too, but he also knows it has a lot of power over him. He can remember when he was a child how he enjoyed wrestling with his younger brothers. He enjoyed pinning them and making them squirm until they said "uncle." He also remembers the hatred he felt toward the "dumb jocks" who were the kings of his high school. He used to fantasize about being strong enough to beat *them* up, about making them cry and feel awe for Ricardo. While many adolescent boys engaged in similar behaviors and created similar fantasies, to Ricardo those memories and impulses are most disturbing. He worries that they indicate something deeply flawed about his character, something that would be let loose if he were to gain physical strength. As you are reading, you may already be developing arguments as to how Ricardo is misinterpreting these memories. Ricardo's friends could also develop similar arguments. But he sees his beliefs as *the truth* about himself, as an accurate view of who he is deep down inside.

He might be right.

But he might be wrong.

When we treat an assumption as if it is the absolute truth, we allow it to rule our actions. We allow it to shape everything we see. We don't consider or explore any other possibilities, and so it continues to hold enormous power over us. That is why it is a ***Big Assumption***. But if and when we are able to name the Big Assumptions underlying our immunities to change, we are able to consider the possibility that they may not actually be 100% true.

Question 5: When you look over all that you have uncovered, and especially your 3rd column commitments, what does that suggest about your assumptions – the beliefs you hold about yourself and how things are – that connect to and support your immune system?

Generate as many Big Assumptions as you can.

Here are a few guidelines for doing this work:

- Some of your Big Assumptions may feel undeniably true ("What do you mean, 'an assumption'? I think this is exactly the awful thing that would happen!"). Some you may know aren't really true (although you act and feel as if they were true); and some you may feel are only partially or sometimes true. **However true you believe your Big Assumptions are, *all of these go in your 4th column***, and will be valuable resources when we turn – in the next chapter – to how you can use your map to help you change.

- ***Every Big Assumption should show why one or more of your hidden commitments feel absolutely necessary.*** If Ricardo were sure there is a dark and untrustworthy part of himself that could be unleashed, then of course he would be committed to not putting himself in a situation (like the gym) where that would be likely to occur. You should be able to follow your map backwards – to see how the Big Assumptions make your third column commitments necessary; how the third column commitments lead to your second column behaviors; and how these behaviors undermine your Column 1 goals. ***Your Big Assumptions set clear limits on what you must do and what you must not do.*** That is, you should be able to see that your Big Assumptions are rules you have for how to live your life, rules you must always follow if you want to avoid danger and disaster and defeat. But you might also be able to see (at least hypothetically) that like any other rule, yours could be broken. Ricardo's rule is that he must not awaken the dark and untrustworthy part of himself that surely exists inside of him. It is a rule he has followed steadfastly, and it might be a good rule, one that is keeping some dangerous impulses caged. But Ricardo can also admit that it might also be possible that his rule could be just a bit flawed. There may be some chance, however slight, that he has overstated the danger, that any dark parts within himself are not going to rise up and take him over, that he can tiptoe a bit closer to this part of himself and check it out to see if it really is as dark and powerful as he thinks it is. And maybe he could gain physical strength and stamina without making any undesirable changes to his character.

- Generate as many Big Assumptions as you can and write them into Column 4 in your map template. Feel free to read ahead before you do so and see what Big Assumptions Miriam, Ron and Maya identified. Some of their entries may resonate with you.

Big Assumptions: Miriam, Ron, and Maya

Miriam looked at her immunity map and could see how her improvement goal (to keeping up better habits) was in complete opposition to her hidden commitment (to staying overweight). She could also see another issue that was connected in some way to being overweight–her feelings about herself. Looking at her third column, she saw that being overweight was connected to being unhappy, to hiding who she really was, what she really wanted, to not being rejected. So what were these connections? Slowly, Miriam began to list them. By the time she had written each item on list, her hand was trembling. She closed her eyes and took several deep breaths.

Miriam

COLUMN 1	COLUMN 2	COLUMN 3	COLUMN 4
My Improvement Goal	"Doing and Not Doing"	Hidden Counter-Commitments	My Big Assumptions
• I'm committed to getting better at creating and following new lifelong food habits – no fad diets, no drastic approaches that I can't keep up.	• I don't keep up healthy eating habits (eat too much fat & sugar; eat big portions; eat snacks). • I set unrealistic goals (e.g., lose 5 pounds in one week). • If I have one slip-up, I use that as an excuse to give up – and then I gorge myself. • I criticize myself really harshly whenever I make a dieting mistake. • I constantly compare myself to thin people who all seem better than me, and then I eat to make myself feel better. • I don't exercise.	Worry box: I fear I will believe I am okay (when I'm clearly not!). I fear I will lose weight and have no excuses, nothing to hide behind. I will be exposed and rejected. • I am committed to not being clueless or blindsided about the ways I am screwed up. • I am committed to not losing being fat as an excuse. • I am committed to hiding behind my weight. • I am committed to not letting up on myself. • I am committed to not letting anyone reject 'the real me.'	• I assume if I don't criticize myself really harshly, I'll slack off too much. • I assume that if I don't criticize myself, others will. • I assume if people saw the real me, they would reject me. • I assume that if I try to lose weight, I will actually feel worse, be under more pressure, and I will fail. • I assume I have even bigger faults than my weight that will keep me unhappy, and if I get thin I will have to face these, and I won't be able to deal with them.

Ron's Big Assumptions were hard for him to identify because they seemed more like facts than beliefs. In Ron's eyes, everyone wants to fit in. There was no alternative for him but to try to be one of the guys. These rules, he felt, were simply the way things are for everyone. Unable to see any other possibilities, he simply reworded his hidden commitments beginning with the words, "I assume..." "I assume I fit in with my friends. I assume I am one of the guys." But again, he felt stuck. He *did* fit in with his friends.

He was one of the guys. Right? The problem was that his friends thought eating healthy was stupid and girly. The problem was that his friends would give him crap if he did try to eat healthy. "I *don't* really fit in. I just pretend I do. So what's my rule or belief, here?" he asked himself. "I guess maybe that I can't find a way to eat better and not get teased. I can't find a way to shut them up."

Ron

COLUMN 1	COLUMN 2	COLUMN 3	COLUMN 4
My Improvement Goal	"Doing and Not Doing"	Hidden Counter-Commitments	My Big Assumptions
• I'm committed to getting better at eating healthier when I'm around other people – at the bar, at parties, at meetings where there is food.	• I eat what my friends eat. • I eat when I am having fun. • I drink too much beer, and then I eat even more. • I don't tell other people I'm trying to lose weight. • When I am talking to people, I don't think about what I am eating. I just keep putting the food in my mouth. • I eat what is on my plate, even if I'm not hungry anymore.	Worry box: I worry that my friends will taunt me about being like a girl. I worry that I'll have to stop hanging out with them completely. I worry that I won't feel like I am part of the group, no matter what they do. • I am committed to fitting in with my friends, to not being one of the "weird guys." • I am committed to not being cast out from the group.	• I assume my friends will tease me if I change the way I eat. • I assume I can't tell my friends to cut it out. • I assume that if I did, they'll think I'm weird. • I assume how I eat with them matters a lot to my friends. • I assume that if I am the weird one, I am not fitting in, I am not one of the guys. • I assume (no matter what my friends do) that I'll feel less a part of things, and that I am missing out on the full experience if I am not eating like my friends are eating.

When Maya admitted to Abigail that her hidden commitments didn't really make sense, she was well on the way to identifying her Big Assumptions. She could see that whenever she rebelled against the advice of books and doctors, she felt that made her right. She could also see that even though that reasoning didn't make a whole lot of sense, she acted as if it did. "I assume I am the only one who is right about me, and that everyone else is wrong," she wrote. The others were easy to identify as well.

Maya

COLUMN 1	COLUMN 2	COLUMN 3	COLUMN 4
My Improvement Goal	"Doing and Not Doing"	Hidden Counter-Commitments	My Big Assumptions
• I'm committed to making better food choices and being more active.	• I buy healthy stuff, but I always keep unhealthy stuff around too. • If I'm out, I'll make an excuse to stop at a convenience store for junk food. • I don't join a gym because I know I won't go. • I keep junk food in my desk at work, and I'll eat that instead of going to get something better. • I watch too much TV. • I drink soda instead of water.	Worry box: I fear spending my life having to follow someone else's rules. I fear being categorized as either a "good" girl or a "bad" girl, depending on what I eat. • I am committed to running my own life, not following someone else's rules. • I'm committed to not giving up control. • •I'm committed to not being the "bad" girl in the dieting world.	• I assume that I am the only one who is right about me, and that everyone else is wrong. • I assume that if I am not making decisions about what to eat, that someone else is running my life. • I assume that I know how to run my own life. • I assume that if I have to stick to a diet or a meal plan, that means I can't control myself.

Alejandra's Story

Alejandra worked for a large public interest law firm and was seen there as a rising star. Now in her mid-thirties, she tended to work long hours and maintain a demanding workload. As a result, she neglected to take care of her health and was starting to notice the results. Over the last ten years, she had gained 35 pounds. She ate poorly and rarely exercised. While she often vowed to work harder on these goals, she found that she was unable to follow through. There was always something happening at work or with her friends that seemed to take priority, derailing her efforts to change her lifestyle. Alejandra was very annoyed and frustrated with herself that she hadn't been able to make any real progress on this area of her life. "It just doesn't fit with how I see myself," she fumed. Everything else in life felt in control – she had always been able to set high goals for herself and then work doggedly until she achieved them. But when it came to food and exercise, it was like she was a different person.

When Alejandra heard about the concept of immunity to change, she immediately saw how this idea might apply to her. Over and over she had made promises to herself to improve her health and fitness, and each time, she broke those promises. Picking up a pencil to draft an ITC map, she knew exactly how to phrase her improvement goal: "I'm committed to prioritizing weight loss by following through on my goals for exercise and better eating." Identifying what she was doing (and also what she was not doing) that undermined her improvement goal was also easy, and Alejandra was aware of how she usually derailed all of her plans to change. She quickly developed her list:

- I eat whatever I want.
- I don't cook for myself.
- I eat whatever food is most convenient to buy and eat – usually fast food.
- I always prioritize commitments I have in my professional life or social life over my health goals.
- If I start to improve my eating and exercise and then have one slip-up, I give up completely and go back to my old unhealthy habits.

But when she turned to her "worry box," she got stuck. Whenever she asked herself what fears would arise if she did cook for herself and if she ate better, she could only think about the benefits. "If I was really careful about my eating, if I were cooking healthy meals for myself instead of grabbing fast food, if I were able to keep the other parts of my life from interfering with my health goals… that would just be great! I'd lose weight, have more energy, feel wonderful!"

She imagined herself cooking some of the meals her mother had made for her when she was a girl.

She thought about how wonderful it would be to feel like she had more control over her life because she wouldn't be constantly starting and stopping new diets. She could picture how good it would feel to be able to wear some of the clothes she wore when she was still in college — clothes that had been sitting in boxes for years now.

Looking for inspiration, Alejandra dragged these boxes of clothes out of her attic, opened them, and pulled out some of the dresses, skirts, and blouses she once wore. As she held them up one at a time to examine them, she was flooded with memories from her college days. She remembered the parties and dances she had gone to, wearing tight, sexy dresses and uncomfortable high heels. She held up a low cut blouse that had been short enough to expose her tummy and trendy belly button ring when she wore it. She laughed when she pulled out a pair of jeans decorated with rivets and embroidery. She remembered that those jeans were so tight that she was uncomfortable when she sat down! "OK, forget that idea! I'll never wear these clothes again!" she laughed, noticing that she felt embarrassed and uncomfortable to remember how she had once dressed. "Even if I do lose weight, I could ***never*** look so trashy... so..." She wasn't sure what word to choose. All she knew was what she felt. **"YUCK!"**

As she piled the clothes back into the boxes as quickly as she could, Alejandra's feeling of "yuck" persisted. She thought about some of the secretaries who dressed in sexy clothes and were always talking about their boyfriends. She thought about some of the women she saw putting on their makeup as they rode the subway each morning and evening. As Alejandra watched these women every day, she often felt annoyed. They seemed so silly and superficial – spending so much energy and attention on how they looked, focusing so much on whether other people would see them as pretty or sexy. The more she thought about these women — and the more she remembered the way she used to dress, and why — the more Alejandra realized that she ***did*** have a worry box. There were good reasons why she wasn't working harder to make sure she ate right and exercised. There were good reasons why she made sure that her work and her friends always came first. To take care of herself by eating and exercising would mean that she would start to look better. And while there was something appealing about looking better, it also felt like a big danger zone. "I've criticized those silly, superficial women because I don't want to be one of them! I don't want to feel that way – so focused on my face, my body, my hair. And I don't want to be seen that way! That's the yuck. That's the thing I fear!"

Alejandra began to write: "I fear that if I focus my energies on food and exercise, that means I overvalue my appearance. I will be vain, petty, self-centered. I am afraid of being only what people see on the surface, of not being taken seriously, not being seen as a person of substance.

I want people to be drawn to my abilities and my mind, not my body." These fears quickly translated into competing commitments.

- I am committed to not seeing myself as or appearing vain, self-centered, or superficial.
- I am committed to not having my abilities and mind discounted.
- I am committed to not making it easier for others to be distracted by my appearance and discount me professionally.

She sat back and looked at what she had written. Now it was all starting to make sense for her. The idea of getting thinner and healthier was so tied up with how she looked and how others reacted to that. The idea of looking better was really complicated – it was appealing but also felt very dangerous. She remembered the ways the guys she knew and even much older men had paid attention to her when she was in college. She thought about how hard she had worked, then and now, to prove to others that she had a good mind, that she was smart and capable and serious and committed. She thought about how it felt to work in an office where the professionals were mostly men. She thought about how angry she got now whenever her family asked whether she was meeting any nice men, whether she was dating anyone, but never had any questions about her work. Slowly, she wrote down:

- I assume that any attention I give to losing weight and to my appearance also gives my approval and support to our cultural overvaluing of how women should look (beauty, femininity, surface-level features), and pulls me into being, and seeming, vain and superficial.

- I assume people (men, especially) will take me less seriously as a professional and a person of substance if I am thinner and more attractive.

For the first time, Alejandra understood why she had let herself become so unhealthy. And for the first time in a long time, she felt some genuine excitement and hopefulness that things were about to change.

Alejandra

COLUMN 1	COLUMN 2	COLUMN 3	COLUMN 4
My Improvement Goal	"Doing and Not Doing"	Hidden Competing-Commitments	My Big Assumptions
• I'm committed to prioritizing weight loss by following through on my goals for exercise and better eating.	• I eat whatever I want. • I don't cook for myself. • I eat whatever food is most convenient to buy and eat – usually fast food • I always prioritize commitments I have in my professional life or social life over my health goals. • If I start to improve my eating and exercise and then have one slip-up, I give up completely and go back to my old unhealthy habits.	Worry box: I fear that if I focus my energies on food and exercise, that means I overvalue my appearance. I will be vain, petty, self-centered. I am afraid of being only what people see on the surface, of not being taken seriously, not being seen as a person of substance. I want people to be drawn to my abilities and my mind, not my body. • I am committed to not seeing myself as or appearing vain, self-centered, or superficial. • I am committed to not having my abilities and mind discounted. • I am committed to not making it easier for others be distracted by my appearance and discount me professionally.	• I assume that any attention I give to losing weight and to my appearance also gives my approval and support to our cultural overvaluing of how women should look (beauty, femininity, surface-level features); and pulls me into being, and seeming, vain and superficial. • I assume people (men, especially) will take me less seriously as a professional and a person of substance if I am thinner and more attractive.

Making Your Map More Powerful

If you have filled in Column 3 (and/or 4) but haven't yet created an immunity map that feels both compelling and intriguing to you, it is worth going back over your answers now to see if you can revise them. Even if your map feels like it packs a punch, you may feel like you want to tinker with it a bit more. Here are our suggestions for how you can make your map stronger:

Column 1: Your Improvement Goal

- Does this column accurately express your hopes? Some people find that they need to push themselves to clarify the ways they describe their improvement goal until it says exactly what they mean.

- Like many of our clients, you may need to focus carefully on the *get better at* part of your improvement goal, in order to zero in on what most needs to change if you are to achieve your goal. Instead of writing, "I am committed to getting better at losing 35 pounds" in Column 1, you may find that there is something more specific you need to improve if you are going to be able to lose that weight. Your improvement goal may then become much better defined: "I am committed to get better at putting down my fork when I'm full."

- Once you have pressed yourself to refine your Column 1 improvement goal, you will be better placed to revise the other columns as well.

Column 2: The Things You Are Doing and Not Doing That Undermine Your Improvement Goal

- Did you list everything you can think of? Did you give yourself lots of time to think? Often we find that when people look at this column again they are able to identify behaviors they didn't think of the first time. If your list is pretty short and/or rather vague, you might want to seek the opinions of others who could offer insight into how you might need to change your behaviors to reach your goal. Think about asking your friends, your family, your doctor, a nutritionist, an exercise coach at the gym, or anyone else who might be well informed about weight loss strategies. Sometimes it can even help to just *imagine* what they might add to your list. If you are following a particular diet and exercise plan, you can also consider its big-picture advice regarding lifestyle changes. What behaviors (that you are not doing) do all of these sources recommend? What do they caution you not to do (that you currently are doing)?

- Are there one or two behaviors that seem to be the biggest obstacles for you? Maybe you do fine all day but then overeat in the evenings. If you could stop doing that, you are sure you'd be able to make significant progress. If there are such behaviors that seem to most get in your way, circle them or underline them to make sure you are paying the most attention to them when you start to think about your fears.

- Then continue on to see if those revisions in Column 2 help you revise Columns 3 and 4.

Column 3: Your Fears and Hidden, Competing Commitments

Column 3 is where folks are most likely to get off-track. It may be the case that you misread one of our directions or suggestions. You may identify fears that are fears about continuing to do the Column 2 behavior. For example, in Column 2 you wrote "I don't exercise much" and then in your Worry Box you entered, "I fear I will get so out of shape I will have health problems." This is a fear about *continuing* the behavior of not exercising. Instead, you need to identify the fear connected with exercising more frequently (the *opposite* of your Column 2 behavior), for example, "I fear I will get my hopes up and then be disappointed when I slack off again." Or you may identify hidden competing commitments that have a kind of noble ring to them, such as, "I am committed to pushing myself to my limits, to expecting more of myself." Or you may come up with something that feels true but also kind of weak and unsurprising, such as, "I am committed to enjoying my meals." Who isn't? If any of these problems is true for you, we suggest you go back over our directions for identifying your fears and hidden, competing commitments to see if that helps you identify something more powerful. Here are some additional suggestions for this important column:

- How powerful do your fears feel? In particular, focus on the behaviors in Column 2 that feel as if they are the biggest obstacles for you and imagine doing the *opposite*. Give yourself more time to think and to imagine, to see what comes up. You may have more than one fear for each behavior. For example, let's imagine your biggest obstacle in Column 2 is something like, "I wait to go to the grocery store or to a restaurant until I am starving, and then I choose the most fattening foods and I overeat." Imagine you were to do the opposite of that. Say you set a particular time to go to the grocery store or to a restaurant, and you made sure to choose a time when you wouldn't be starving. *What fears or worries would come up for you*? Maybe the first one that comes to mind is a worry that following such a schedule would be less convenient. OK, but that worry is pretty manageable. Is there more to it than that? Ask yourself, "What would be the *worst* thing about following that schedule?" When you push yourself to consider this possibility further and fan the fire of your worries, you may come to something deeper. "I fear I would lose my sense of freedom and spontaneity." Or, "I fear that I'll feel deprived." Or, "I fear that I'll feel empty – in my stomach *and* in my spirit."

- When you translate your fears to hidden, competing commitments, make sure you preserve the sense of danger in your wording. Sometimes the power of the fear gets bleached out, and you may need to reword your commitment so that it captures that danger. If you fear that your mother will feel deeply hurt when you don't eat her lasagna, but your hidden commitment is to "showing how much I love my mother," you've lost something in translation. How about, "I am committed to not losing the role of 'good son' my mother expects me to be and to not having her feel I have left her behind?" Or, "I am committed to avoiding any possibility of discord in our family, at all costs?"

- Experiment with slightly different wording and different versions of the same idea. "I am committed to expecting more of myself" may be the noble way of expressing a scarier but more powerful feeling, such as, "I am committed to not feeling like a quitter or a failure." If you've got one that feels "blah" to you, such as "I am committed to enjoying my meals," see if you can press yourself harder on that one too. What was the fear in the worry box that led you to this? If it was revulsion for bland or mass-produced, microwavable "diet food," how about "I am committed to not having to eat disgusting food," or "I'm committed to not losing all the joy from eating"? Our list of common fears and hidden commitments (at the end of chapter 2) can also give you some ideas.

Column 4: Your Big Assumptions

Having trouble identifying the Big Assumptions that keep your whole immune system in place? These can be hard for us to see if we can't imagine that things could be any different than how we have been thinking about them.

- Big Assumptions often involve ideas about what we absolutely *can't do* or *shouldn't do*. ("I assume that if I try to lose weight, I will fail, and then I will feel worse than I do now." "I assume if I do eat more healthily, my husband won't like what I cook and will be annoyed with me.") Or they may involve what we feel we *must do* ("I assume that I always have to be the one who helps others reach their goals."). Look at your map to see if there are any places you seem to be thinking along these lines and consider whether you might be making some Big Assumptions.

- Big Assumptions can also lurk whenever we see things in stark terms. If there is something that feels very black-and-white, like it is *either* all one way *or* all another way, you may actually be overstating things in a way that suggests you are making a Big Assumption. For example, if my improvement goal is to "find the beautiful, slim me that I dream of," and one of my fears is that I will fail and "see that I will always be ugly and fat," I've only given myself two options: a wonderful one and a horrible one. What are my assumptions? Perhaps they are: "I assume that if I don't follow my diet perfectly, and I screw up even once, then I might as well give up and admit that I'll never succeed." Or, "I assume that thin people are morally good and deserve to be happy and overweight people are morally bad and deserve to be unhappy."

- Big Assumptions are often distortions, and the three most common distortions (per Martin Seligman in *Learned Optimism*, we call them "PER thinking") are:

    - over-PERsonalizing ("I assume if my husband gets angry with me I *must* be doing something wrong.")

    - overly PERsistent, a "time" distortion ("I assume if he is angry with me *now* he will be angry *forever*.")

    - overly PERvasive, a "spatial" distortion ("I assume if my husband gets angry with me, *my in-laws will also get angry*, and pretty *soon the whole family will be angry with me*."

The idea, at the moment, is not to *correct* any of this thinking but just to identify that you may hold some Big Assumptions that partake in these distortions.

If you succeeded in generating some Big Assumptions for yourself, we are soon going to show you that you have *also* found the keys to overturning your immune system, the keys to losing weight and/or keeping it off. Maybe you didn't take our advice earlier about engaging this chapter like a workbook. We understand that sometimes it can feel better to know where something is heading before doing it. But at this point, to get the most out of this book—and to accomplish your health goal—you now need to actually create your own immunity map in order to really understand the radical idea in this book about how to change. Once you develop your own immunity map, you should now see a whole new vista for change opening up before you. You may still feel uncertain as to *how* you can move into this new space, as to how it can actually help you – and that is just what we will turn to next.

PART TWO

Exploring Where You Are Now

Before we put you to work overturning your immunities, we want to share with you a little bit about how this process happens and what makes it work. The map below depicts the dynamic equilibrium of the immune system and its countervailing forces; working with one foot on the gas and one foot on the brakes.

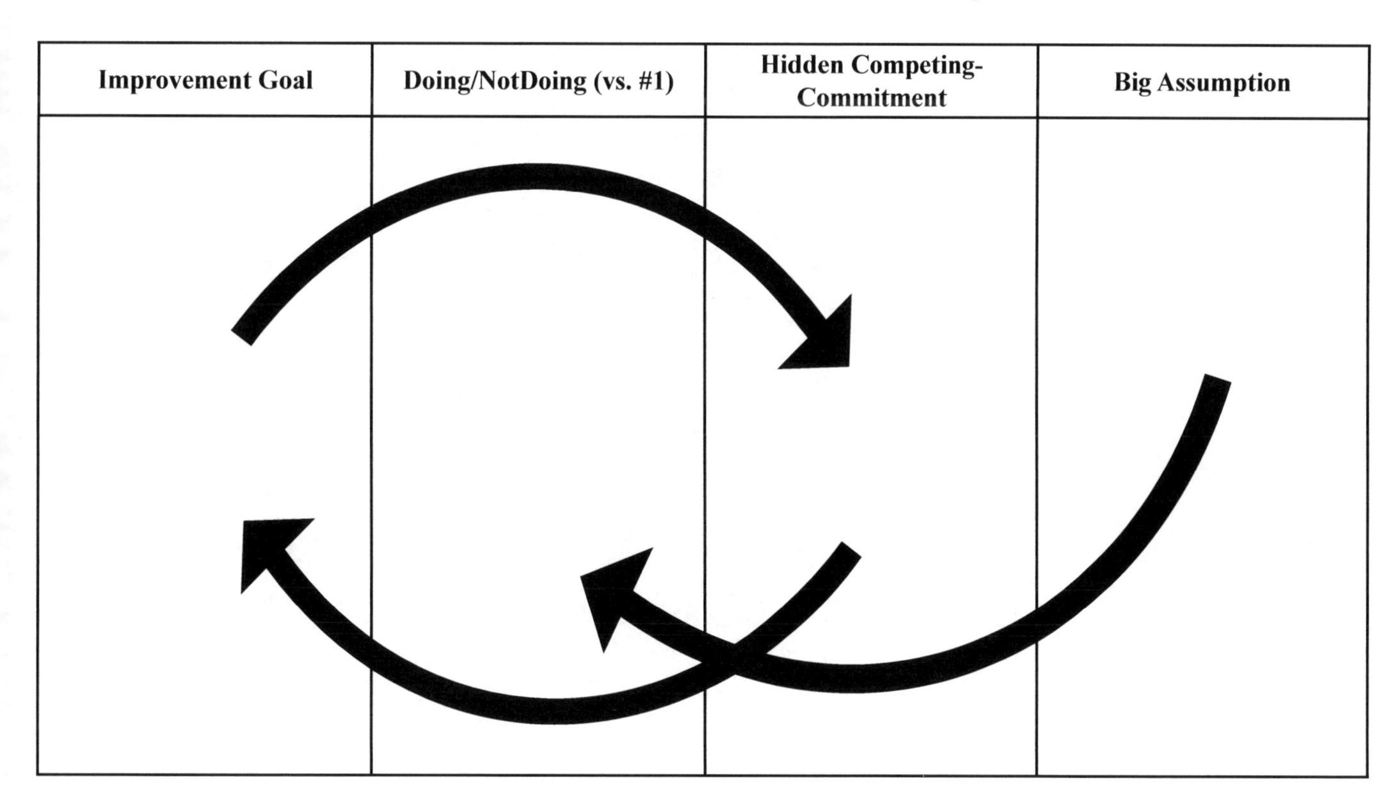

When you are immune, your Big Assumptions are the things keeping that immunity in place, keeping the Column 1 and Column 3 arrows working directly against each other, tying you into a knot. The way to loosen or even untie the Column 1-Column 3 knot is to release the pressure on it. That pressure comes from the Big Assumptions. Your Big Assumptions are what keeps your immune system in place. They are what keep the pressure on that immunity knot.

The pressure our Big Assumptions place on us comes from the roles they have played for us – as rules we are either unaware of or believe are 100% true, all of the time, if we are to stay safe. The best way to release some of the pressure is therefore to bring them in front of us, to call them into question, to begin to raise doubts about them, so as to understand them better – to learn when they are right and when they are wrong, when they are useful to us and when they interfere.

4

Recognizing Obstacles: Start With Your BAs

I used to set myself up for failure. I used to put myself in situations where I would get hurt. But I deserve better. When I started this process, I just felt like I was going to have a life-altering experience. But I really can't believe how things lined up, how things happened as they did. Maybe I just needed to be ready. I had assumed that if I really tried to deal with the stuff that was holding me back, I wouldn't be able to. It would lead to bad consequences for everyone. But I stood up for myself, and I took some risks to figure things out. I feel like no matter what happens, I will be OK. I will make the best decisions I can. I feel like I can love myself.

— *Andrea*

Why are Big Assumptions so powerful and so difficult to question? Our Big Assumptions often seem as though they are necessary for survival on our journey through life. They tell us things like where we think there is danger or disaster, where there is something completely unknown, where we will feel the awful sense that we are powerless, out of control, vulnerable, alone, or isolated. The problem is that they may not be right. They are screaming "Warning! Warning!" to us, but we may find that they are like overprotective pet dogs who are convinced that everyone who approaches the house is a danger. While they may keep the house and its occupants safe, they also prevent friends from entering too.

The dog "assumes" that *everyone* intends to harm us, that *everyone* presents a threat, that there is never any alternative but to snarl, lunge, and attack. That assumption may work well if you specifically want a watchdog who will stop at nothing to protect your property, but it creates all kinds of problems if the dog lives in your house, and you actually like to have guests! Your dog (just like a Big Assumption) is often mistaken, but it is just trying to take good care of you. We don't need to shoot the dog or the person at the door. We can appreciate this loyal intention, and we can also learn to question the dog's alarm. We can consider who should be running things, the dog or the owner? We can take a look out the window and decide for ourselves, "Is there really a dangerous intruder at the door, or is it just the friendly mailman?"

Sometimes, people can look at their maps and know – intellectually – that their Big Assumptions are not true. One person had the Big Assumption that "I assume that when I am stressed out, I will feel better if I indulge in junk food (especially ice cream)." After writing down this Big Assumption, she said, "I can tell you right now, that's not true for more than the minute I'm eating it. I never feel better after I indulge. I usually feel worse because I've proved to myself, once again, that I am greedy and weak-willed. I actually feel *ashamed*. But I still *act* as if I believe I am going to feel better — if I'm stressed, I will automatically eat. I can't seem to learn that it doesn't help."

Other times, people feel like their Big Assumptions are 100% accurate — that they will never learn to overturn them because they shouldn't. They are actually correct. For example, one person who successfully overturned her immunity and lost all the weight she had hoped to reflected back on how pessimistic she had felt when she began the work.

> "When I look back I wonder how it could have gone on so long. I have to say I'm shocked. When we first started, I thought "there is no way I can change" because I had done it this way for so long. I think I was a little bit nervous when we first started. I didn't quite get how this was going to be different from other things I've tried. I've tried Weight Watchers and Nutrisystem. I took all these classes on self-esteem. And when I wrote down my Big Assumptions, I didn't believe I would ever change them. I remember you said I would, and that just didn't make any sense to me at all. I thought, "How is *that* going to happen?" I really thought that my beliefs were actually just the way things were."

Understanding your Big Assumptions allows you to make deeper and better distinctions between the situations when you need to protect yourself and those when you are over-protecting and creating problems for yourself. The more accurately we understand our Big Assumptions, the less we will feel unnecessary fear and alarm. The less we feel unnecessary fear and alarm, the more the second column behaviors change. The more the second column behaviors change, the more you fulfill your goal – permanently, because you are getting your mind "right" before getting your weight right. The exercises that appear here are designed to help you understand your Big Assumptions better. They will help you to safely explore territory that has come to feel so dangerous in order to grow more comfortable with it.

We now invite you to journey with us through an exploration of your own Big Assumptions that can lead you to feel quite differently about them. If you are willing to do this work your Big Assumptions will no longer have you in their grip, holding you tightly knotted, preventing you from making progress on your improvement goals. If you are willing to do this work, you will begin to find new feelings of relaxation, spaciousness, choice, and freedom that come with seeing your Big Assumptions more clearly and accurately, creating new possibilities for your life.

All of the exercises that follow are tools you can use to navigate your journey as nimbly as possible. Think of them as maps and compasses and binoculars and signs – all of the markers and guides we have learned are useful for people who set out on these journeys and reach their destination. These tools are also important because they help us maintain a certain type of stance or attitude toward our journey. They are designed to help you to be more objective, open, friendly, and curious toward yourself so you can learn as much as possible about the accuracy of your Big Assumptions. They are designed to help you steer away from some of the inner obstacles (self-criticism, inhibition, fear, judgment) that could get in your way.

It may help to frame your work in overturning your immunities by imagining that somebody has hired you to find out as much as possible about some Big Assumptions—the ones you just happen to hold! Your insider perspective will be very useful in developing a reliable route to take in reaching your goals. What you learn will be very important as it may change not only your own life but also those of countless others who face similar predicaments with their weight. Think of yourself as a kind of researcher (a scientist, an explorer, an anthropologist, even an astronaut if it helps)—a trailblazer doing advance work for yourself and for those who will follow.

What we are going to ask you to do over the next several weeks may at first feel difficult because you haven't done it before, but we have a few words of encouragement:

- It will get easier as you get accustomed to this kind of work, and as you begin to see and feel something new.

- Getting your mind "right" provides its own boost and sense of progress, so you won't need your goal to be accomplished to acquire the confidence that you are getting somewhere and to give you the energy to stay the course.

- The exercises we are going to ask you to do are not forever. The mind shift will last, but will eventually take care of itself.

- It works, if you do.

You'll need to follow exacting standards and study these BAs very carefully – proceeding systematically, developing your interpretations carefully, relying strictly on "data" and evidence, considering and exploring alternative explanations. You'll have to study all obstacles and dead end tracks, and document your findings thoroughly. Like most good explorers, you'll want to go slow so you can go far. That is the only way to be sure that the conclusions you draw and the routes you choose are as accurate as possible.

The reason we suggest you imagine yourself as a researcher/explorer is to invite you to be more aware for a while of what you are thinking, feeling, and doing than most of us typically are. If you approach your familiar surroundings as suddenly strange or foreign in order to describe and explain them to someone who has never been there, you will no longer be following your established patterns of thinking and behavior. You might become more curious and more open to seeing with new eyes, noticing patterns you've never seen before. Along the way, new questions and new reflections will emerge. You should develop a researcher/explorer's disciplined approach – a careful, systematic, responsible, detailed way of building solid foundations for your journey of learning and change.

The exercises that follow are designed to call upon all these skills. In the same way that the immunity-to-change map led you carefully to new insights about yourself, these exercises can help you try on and evaluate different ways of thinking about yourself and different ways of behaving—ways of overturning the immunities you uncovered in your ITC map. They are designed to keep you in the "sweet spot" where insight-leading-to-new-action is most likely to happen – when you are feeling open, aware, and curious.

Change Your Beliefs To Change Your Behaviors

Early in this book, we explained our belief that for most of you, reaching and maintaining a healthy weight requires changing not only your behavior but your mind. When you diagnosed your immunity to change you identified the specific beliefs (your Big Assumptions) that need to change, along with your behavior, if you are to lose weight and keep it off

We remind you of this idea here because as you begin to work to overturn your immunities, you may find yourself paying attention to your behaviors (what you eat and don't eat) and to results (the number on the scale, or the measurement of your waistline) and paying less attention to what is happening with the Big Assumptions that have played a big part in causing your problems in the first place. ***So keep in mind: because those beliefs are the source of your worst problems, you will only be able to make sustainable change by addressing and changing them.***

Don't worry. The work you are about to do is not extraordinarily difficult. We have seen hundreds of people just like you use this approach to successfully make changes that seemed impossible before. We will keep reminding you to focus on your Big Assumptions, and we'll show you many different ways that you can be working on them. Later, we'll invite you to make some very specific and important changes to your behavior as a way to test your BAs. We'll ask you to observe yourself, to develop a vision for your success, and to uncover the origins of your BAs. To complete these exercises, you'll need to behave differently than you normally do, but as you'll see, we are not yet asking you to change how or what or when you eat. We are not asking you to change how much or how little you exercise. Nor are we asking you to weigh yourself more often or less often than you have been doing up until now. We actually won't ask you to make such changes until the end of the book. You may be eager to forge ahead, but there is a danger in doing so before you've addressed your BAs.

The danger is that when you try to change your behavior, you may end up repeating the patterns of the past: relying on a combination of will power and self-discipline to try to change your lifestyle; triggering the same commitments and assumptions that have kept you immune, and then when you don't see the progress you were hoping for, feeling worse about yourself and giving up. We think this danger is particularly relevant for people with long histories of losing weight, only to regain it again.

However, we are not going to *forbid* you to make changes in your eating and exercise habits. Often, even when we beg for patience from the people we work with in person (when we can be fooled into thinking we have more influence), they go out and start making changes anyway. We explain our reasoning and offer our cautions, and they nod their heads because they can see that we are making a lot of sense. But it doesn't stop them from jumping right in.

We try not to take their actions personally. We get it. They're excited. They feel so motivated. They are starting to learn what has gone wrong in the past. And they almost can't hold themselves back. Maybe you're feeling that way too?

You may already be making plans for or getting started on the changes you think you'll need to make. Maybe you have joined a weight loss program or a new gym. Maybe you have starting buying healthier food, or cooking with healthier ingredients, or making and bringing a healthier lunch to work. Maybe you bought this book (or someone gave it to you) because you have already started a new diet or exercise regimen and you hope this will boost your chances of success. That's all right. If you think you have some reasonable and safe ideas for changing your eating and exercise habits, we suggest you stop reading this chapter and skip over to Chapter 8, Designing Tests. That chapter will help you think about how to make safe and modest changes – *not* to see whether you can successfully alter your eating and exercise habits – and not to see if the number on the scale will go lower – but ***to see what you can learn about your Big Assumptions.*** Huh? Don't know what we mean by that? Good! Go read the chapter. Then you can come back and work on these exercises while you are also designing and running your tests.

Are some of you still here? We hope so! We want to congratulate you on wisely deciding to delay making changes to your behavior. And we also want to let you know that by delaying, you are by no means taking an easy way through this work. For many, the exercises that follow will be hard but rewarding work. You'll learn plenty. And these exercises will take you to the point where you will be much more ready to begin to change your eating and exercise behaviors as well. For those of you who are coming back to this chapter after having skipped ahead, welcome back! These exercises will provide you with other ways (in addition to testing) to think differently about and work through your Big Assumptions.

As we continue to follow the stories of Miriam and Ron, you'll notice that Miriam began to make changes to her eating habits right away. She was careful to start slowly and with the help of a reputable weight loss program, like Weight Watchers, and a nutritionist. However, Ron felt more comfortable postponing any of these behavioral changes. It wasn't until he began to run tests of his Big Assumptions that he started trying to change the ways that he ate at all.

How Will You Know You're Making Progress?

It is easy to think that completing these exercises will automatically overturn your BAs. If you start from this perspective, you will want to move quickly through each exercise, answering our questions, putting text in the the columns, and checking off that exercise so that you can move on to the next one, with the goal of being able to check that one off too... until you're "done," right? From that stance, when we suggest that you go back to an earlier exercise (which we often do) you can feel like you are not making progress, as if you are being held back because you didn't do something correctly the first time. You may begin to feel impatient and frustrated by going back and want to keep moving ahead so that you can be "cured."

We suggest that you try *not* to adopt that stance because it often interferes with the type of deep learning that you can experience in this process. The nature of overturning immunities is not like driving down a straight, flat road, moving directly from where you started to where you want to go. Instead, your path might be more like a rock-strewn, barely marked trail up a steep mountain. If you chart a course that leads in a straight line from the bottom to the top, you won't make it. You will tire. You will run smack into obstacles you can't overcome. You will completely miss seeing, understanding, and learning about most of the mountain. And perhaps most importantly, you probably won't make it to the top anyway. Or, we should say, you may make it to the top of the "done with the exercises" mountain but not the "right mind/right weight" mountain. Which one do you want to stand atop?
Because the goal isn't just to complete the exercises. The goal is to overturn your immunity so as to remove the obstacles that block your path to success. To get to the top of that mountain will require a different kind of journey. You may need to "switch back." Switching back means, yes, you will be reversing directions. But you will be reversing directions at a higher level of the mountain than where you were previously. You may see the same parts of the mountain you saw earlier, but you will see them from a new height. You will be gaining ground by working at a sustainable and safe pace. You will be exploring all of the parts of the mountain as you go, learning that territory well, making wise decisions about how to proceed. And that is how you will best find your own way, get to the top, and know thoroughly the route you have taken. That is how you will succeed.

The exercises we invite you to practice are more like habits than steps to complete. You can choose any imagery you like to help you stick to the work: like a musician who still begins every practice by doing scales, or a ballet dancer who begins to dance every day by doing the simple barre exercises she learned as a small child, we return to them often because they are foundational, even as we add to a repertoire (and get better at the ones we learned first). They are the best way we know of to get you up your mountain.

You should also know that people often overturn their immunities without completing every exercise. They always create ITC maps. And they always run tests. But it is not uncommon for clients to skip one of the other exercises in the process when they don't understand it, have a strong aversion to it, or feel stuck about how to complete it. If you are really resisting an exercise, so much so that you lose momentum, skip it and go on. You can always return to it later if you change your mind. You may have one foot on the gas and one on the brake, but *you are* the one in the driver's seat! Ready? Off we go...!

5

PRACTICING SELF-OBSERVATION

I'm getting better at handling stress. When I have time to think, I ask "what's the worst that could happen?" Probably nothing. So I let it go. Before I would just assume that something really bad was going to happen. When I think about it, I see it's not a big deal. You know... say my kids go to the dentist a week late. So what? Before, as soon as something would come up, I would assume it's not good. I realize now when I'm doing that. I can slow that process down. I can cut it off before I get to that point. A friend talked me into doing this program, and I'm glad. Because it actually has changed my life. I have lost weight, and my health improved. My stress reduction has really improved. Now, I've just gotten better at seeing these things coming and talking to myself. Instead of trying to over-prepare and control everything, it feels like it will be OK. It is what it is. If it is something I can do something about, I will. When I handle stress better, I cut back. I am not overwhelmed. I can take care of myself, eat better, feel better.

— Jeri

One of the most important habits for you to practice throughout the entire ITC process is self-observation. What does it mean to be observing yourself? It means that you are watching not only your behaviors, but the ways you think and feel about food, exercise, and weight loss. In these moments, part of you is doing the kinds of things you do every day (overeating at dinner, making an excuse not to go to the Zumba class you enrolled in, buying unhealthy food when you go the supermarket), and another part of you is sort of standing aside and watching yourself. The typical ways we go about our day-to-day lives may be automatic, unconsciously mechanical – we have solidified our routines. The goal of self-observation is to become more conscious of your typical and routine reactions, paying more attention to what you do, why, and with what results.

But, as you will see, we have a very specific approach to "self-observation." It is not just about trying to observe everything, or even everything related to food or weight. We are going to train you to become better observers of your Big Assumptions. If it helps, think of these exercises as collecting information that you will need to interpret and report to someone to help someone make sense of your Big Assumptions.

The Self-Observation Exercises

You may have already done some self-observation when you were filling out your ITC map. For example, in order to identify the types of behaviors that undermine your improvement goal (the behaviors you listed in Column 2), you may have been paying more attention to the things you actually do and don't do. As you observed yourself, you may have noticed the specific things that are your trouble spots (such as eating at night or eating more when you visit your mom). You may have become more aware of the things you don't do that you should (such as taking the stairs instead of the elevator at work). And, of equal importance, you may have noticed the ways that you think or talk to yourself that get in your way (such as when you criticize yourself by calling yourself a "slob" or a "failure").

You may also have been observing yourself to identify the fears, worries, hidden commitments, and Big Assumptions you listed in your map. For example, on Wednesday morning, you may have noticed that you were eating more than you had been eating earlier in the week and recognized that the donuts and bagels that are provided at every Wednesday morning meeting are hard for you to resist. Remembering the ITC map you had been working on, you could then ask yourself, "So, what if I were to get up and move that platter of food to the side of the room, so that the donuts and bagels are not on the table in front of us all? What uneasiness arises for me as I sit here and imagine doing that right now?" The ability to observe yourself can lead to some pretty amazing insights as you come to see yourself more clearly and understand your feelings and ideas more deeply.

If you haven't been engaging in this kind of self-observation up to now, we urge you to start making it a habit. And now that you have read our description of how observations can be so helpful, you may begin to notice additional entries you can make to Columns 2, 3, and 4 of your own ITC map. (Remember what we said in the last chapter about "switching back" in order to forge ahead?)

Now we want to offer some explicit directions about how to observe yourself as you begin to overturn your immunities. To help focus your observations, it helps to know what you will be looking for. That's why we recommend that you choose just one Big Assumption as the focus for now. Sometimes you'll have a few Big Assumptions that are very intertwined with each other so that focusing on one almost inevitably means that you'll be including the others as well. That's fine. Other times the Big Assumptions may be more diverse and unrelated. If that's the case for you, look back at your map and see if you can find one that feels like it is holding you back the most. If you were really able to change one of your Big Assumptions, which one seems like it would make the most difference in overturning your immunity?

Question 1: Look at your list of Big Assumptions. Are there one or two that feel like they are the most powerful for you? Choose the one you want to focus on and enter it into your Change Journal (see page CJ-6).

Take the next week and try to notice all of the situations you face where your Big Assumption is at work, shaping how you think and feel as well as what you do. Again, we recommend that you *not* try to change any of your behaviors or your thinking, tempting though that may be. For now we hope you are still just observing. You might want to plan ahead and identify the types of situations that you're likely to face in the next week or two where your BA might be likely to be in play. For example, if you know you are going to be visiting your in-laws, where food is often plentiful and where you usually eat more than you intend, make a point to observe yourself in that setting. If you weigh yourself regularly on Monday mornings, pay special attention to whether and how your Big Assumption may be relevant to how you think and feel when you stand on the scale.

So what form should these observations take? What should you actually do? Ask yourself the following question:

Question 2: How is my Big Assumption getting in my way in these situations?

In other words, can you notice when your Big Assumption has led you to do things like those you listed in Column 2 of your ITC map that undermine your Column 1 goal?

Try to identify at least four or five such situations and describe each one in the left hand column of the following chart in your Change Journal (p. CJ-7). Write what happened as well as what you were thinking and feeling.

Self-Observation Template

Describe the situations when your Big Assumption got in the way of your improvement goal (including your thoughts & feelings).	**When it got in your way, what specific problems or negative results did your Big Assumption cause you?**
Situation #1:	Situation #1:
Situation #2:	Situation #2:
Situation #3:	Situation #3:
Situation #4:	Situation #4:
Situation #5:	Situation #5:

After you have collected a few observations, read over your description of each situation you wrote about in the left hand column. For each situation, ask yourself these questions: **When you think about what happened, do you see any ways that your Big Assumption was not helping you but instead actually caused you problems? In what ways did your Big Assumption lead to something bad or prevent something good from happening?** Describe these in the right hand column.

Ron's Observations

Ron looked at his list of Big Assumptions:

- I assume my friends will tease me if I change the way I eat.
- I assume I can't tell my friends to cut it out.
- I assume that if I did, they'll think I'm weird.
- I assume how I eat with them matters a lot to my friends.
- I assume that if I am the weird one, I am not fitting in, I am not one of the guys.
- I assume (no matter what my friends do) that I'll feel less a part of things and that I am missing out on the full experience if I am not eating like my friends are eating.

Ron realized that when he made his map, he had focused mostly on one group of his close friends. While he also saw that the assumptions he had listed were closely related, he decided to observe for the last assumption ("no matter what my friends do I'll feel less a part of things and that I am missing out on the full experience if I am not eating like my friends are eating"). As soon as he began to observe himself, he realized that these same assumptions applied to many other relationships such as those he had with work colleagues. They even applied to some acquaintances such as restaurant employees! In the course of one week, Ron observed three key situations when his Big Assumptions guided his choices about when and how much to eat and drink.

Ron's Big Assumption: I assume no matter what my friends do I'll feel less a part of things and that I am missing out on the full experience if I am not eating like my friends are eating.

Ron's Self Observations:

Describe the situations when your Big Assumption got in the way of your improvement goal (including your thoughts & feelings).	When it got in your way, what specific problems or negative results did your Big Assumption cause you?
We go out to eat as a family – usually go to the same restaurant. The owners know me. They know what I like and really enjoy suggesting a new appetizer we should try or new deal on dessert. I feel like they want me to eat a lot too. It's like I'm the guy who likes their food. It makes me feel good that they know me, that they make me feel a part of things.	On one hand, I like being the guy who likes their food and is known there. I don't like that I can't eat whatever I want anymore. But that's true now, and so now I'm the fat guy who eats too much. That's not so good.
Went out with the guys last night. I ate and drank whatever I wanted – more than they did. I felt I was a part of things and that felt good.	I woke up with a hangover and felt tired all day. I don't know why I have to eat and drink the most of anybody.
Birthday party at work for Janice. She brought in a fabulous homemade cake. My favorite kind so I ate two pieces. Everybody knows what kind of cake I like, what kind of food I like. It's not like it was my birthday. So then I ate the cake, and I talked about how great it was. I feel like people want me to do that, like I'd disappoint them if I didn't make a fuss. I felt like I was in the "in" crowd.	It kind of makes me mad-- it's not like they are going to get fatter, so I have to eat the cake. I mean, the cake is good, but sometimes I feel like they don't even give me a choice.

Miriam's Observations

Miriam looked at the list of her Big Assumptions and decided the one that was holding her back the most was:

- I assume if I don't criticize myself really harshly, I'll slack off too much.

She then spent two weeks observing herself to see when this Big Assumption was shaping her decisions and the ways she was interpreting her experiences. Miriam identified several situations (#1-#4). Because she was trying to learn from observing her Column 2 behaviors, she also discovered lots of occasions when she overate that had nothing to do with that Big Assumption. She decided she would enter those into her journal to see if she could figure out what was going on. What she discovered was a new assumption: "I assume that every time I feel stressed or emotional, I must eat to make myself feel better" (#1, #4 - #6).

Miriam's Big Assumption: I assume if I don't criticize myself harshly, I'll slack off too much.

Miriam's Self Observations:

Describe the situations when your Big Assumption got in the way of your improvement goal (including your thoughts & feelings).	When it got in your way, what specific problems or negative results did your Big Assumption cause you?
I had several stressful days and have been making some bad food choices. Haven't exercised at all. I made and ate cookies yesterday. I criticized myself for all of it.	I gained a few pounds. I felt crappy – physically and mentally. I beat myself up.
I was having lunch at a Mexican restaurant with my best friend Ellen. They gave us chips and salsa, which we weren't really eating. After we were already done with our meal, we were still talking, and I started to eat the chips. I don't know why I was doing it. I just ate one but then kept eating more and more – very quickly – until suddenly the basket was empty!! I ate ALL of them!!! I felt horrible, physically and emotionally.	Once I start eating, there's a part of me that knows I'm doing something stupid and sabotaging my plans. Sometimes I feel like I want to hurt myself. Maybe I'm not good enough to be thin and healthy, like I don't deserve it. I criticize my lack of self-discipline. But somehow I think criticizing myself will help me the next time. Weird.

Miriam's Self Observations continued:

Describe the situations when your Big Assumption got in the way of your improvement goal (including your thoughts & feelings).	**When it got in your way, what specific problems or negative results did your Big Assumption cause you?**
Several times, I noticed that I was feeling tired at work and wanted to eat. There are many work-related things which I have on my plate to finish. I am feeling out of control. My stomach has been hurting. I tried not to eat junk, but I was so tired, that I cannot convince myself. Then we had a meeting where I was given more work without any acknowledgement of how much I have already been doing. I could imagine Paul complaining to me again, and I felt hopeless and stressed and lonely. After the meeting, I began eating. I felt no energy to make good choices. I felt no desire to make good choices.	My mood leads me to eat. I eat to feel better, and I eat to celebrate feeling happy. Eating doesn't really help my mood – in fact, I just felt more stressed and more out of control and thinking that I am such an idiot to be stuck in this pattern. I used the self-criticism to get me going though. Once I dug into my work, I started to feel better until it was time to go home, and I hadn't finished enough of it, and I knew I couldn't stay late. Then I felt like crap again.
In yoga class, there are mirrors all around. I started out relaxed, and then I noticed one of my fat rolls, and from there it was downhill. I became fixated on all the things I don't like about my body, all the things that are not the way I want them to be. I felt like quitting right there and then. But then I tried to look at the floor instead of the mirror. I tried not to look up until class was over so I could put on my baggy sweats. As soon as I was out, I headed straight for my chocolate stash.	I have to work really hard to keep from criticizing myself. I could do it for a while, but then I caved in and ate a ton of chocolate. So I had new reason to be self-critical. It's exhausting whether I criticize myself or keep from criticizing myself!!
Paul (my husband) told me he thinks the extra hours I'm putting in at work are negatively impacting the kids. As soon as he said this, I started thinking he's right to criticize me. I felt blindsided. And I proceeded to eat basically the entire big bag of M & Ms.	I feel guilty. I love my job and love that I'm being given extra responsibility there. But then I feel like I'm being a bad wife and mom. I immediately start to think Paul is right to criticize me. I feel like he sees everything that is wrong with me. I hate this feeling and want to eat as a way to make that bad feeling go away.

Miriam's Self Observations continued:

Describe the situations when your Big Assumption got in the way of your improvement goal (including your thoughts & feelings).	**When it got in your way, what specific problems or negative results did your Big Assumption cause you?**
I had a disagreement with my daughter, and I felt like she was judging me. I got very defensive and felt like I had to justify myself and pick at her, show her how she was all to blame. I felt terrible, like I couldn't stand to feel so terrible, couldn't stand to be in my body, to be myself and went right to the kitchen. I grabbed some ice cream from the freezer and a spoon, and just started shoveling it into my mouth. But as I was eating, I thought to myself, "This ice cream is so cold, my tongue has gone numb. I can't even taste what I'm eating." I also thought about how disgusted I would feel later and how poorly I would sleep. But still I kept eating because I was just so angry at myself. Then I could hear Paul coming down the hall towards the kitchen. In a complete panic, I dropped the spoon into the ice cream container and shoved it all back into the freezer. I dreaded him seeing me so out of control.	I felt like a terrible mom and so guilty for yelling at her. Once again, I feel bad and then overeat. Then I feel bad about eating. Ugh. It is so hard to see this about myself – how insecure and silly I am. I wish I didn't have to do this. It's a lot of effort. It's more than I can cope with. I'm not doing as well as I was when I first started. I get really consumed by this and I can't turn it off. Sometimes, I'm overwhelmed and I can't take it. I do feel like there's something I am dealing with emotionally but not necessarily consciously. I feel like my life has been stalled for so long. I'm stuck in a rut. Being upset about the disagreement, about feeling guilty, about feeling like a bad mom, about overeating, and that sugar all meant that I didn't sleep well at all that night. That next morning, I felt more exhausted than when I went to bed. When I heard Paul coming, I could barely contain my panic because I felt so terrified and ashamed. I hadn't even had a chance to beat myself up about it; how could I face him?

So what is the point of this sometimes painful or scary exercise? Not to help you immediately accomplish your goal, obviously. The point is that you are beginning to build muscles that will help you to see how your Big Assumption influences you. The more you look at (rather than through) your assumptions, the more you have *a new relationship* to your assumptions, rather than being *unmindfully run* by them. Remember your barking dog? The one who automatically thinks there really is some danger at the door? We said the first step to putting yourself in charge (vs. your dog) is noticing that the barking creates an opportunity to observe and question, rather than immediately to go into action. Your Big Assumption is your barking dog.

Observing Yourself in Situations That Cast Doubt on Your Big Assumptions

If you are challenged by the idea of observing yourself, you probably want to keep working on the previous exercise before you move to this next one. If you are getting the hang of self-observations and feel ready to try something a little harder, you might want to conduct these next observations at the same time.

In this part of the exercise, you will be looking for **any situations that arise that could indicate that your Big Assumption is not 100% true.** Remember, in order for your findings to be useful, you want to be as thorough as possible, looking for all kinds of relevant information about these Big Assumptions. Looking for evidence that contradicts your Big Assumption doesn't mean you should deliberately do things differently to see what will happen. The only thing you should do differently is pay more attention. Look deliberately and specifically for these types of situations. Again, you might want to plan ahead and identify the types of situations that you're likely to face in the next week or so where your BA might be in play. As you observe yourself, ask yourself the following question:

Question 3: In the next week or so, can I find any situation where I can see (or even imagine) that my BA might possibly be (at least sometimes) *wrong*?

Here are some examples you might find if you look really hard:

- I don't follow my own BA, and it's OK.
- Someone else doesn't seem to have my BA and so behaves as if it is not 100% true and it's OK.
- I do follow my own BA, but I also see a possibility that I might choose not to and that could lead to different results.

We call these types of observations "counter observations" because they are situations that contradict (or run counter to) what our Big Assumptions tell us. You may discover that it is hard for you to recognize these situations because we tend to see only what we are expecting to see, ignoring any information that doesn't agree with what we already think and feel. This is called "confirmation bias." A common example of confirmation bias occurs when thousands of people read the same, one-paragraph horoscope in the newspaper and think that paragraph accurately predicts what kind of day they will have. If a person already believes in astrology, he or she will go through the day only paying attention to the ways that the horoscope correctly forecast what would happen and ignoring any possibilities for how the forecast could have been incorrect. Another common example of confirmation bias occurs when people choose to watch only the cable news channel that aligns with their own political beliefs and only talk politics with people who hold the same views that they do. Interacting only with information and perspectives that support your own views allows you to screen out any opportunities to see other views as valid.

As you observe, remember: ***do not intentionally change anything you do or think that relates to your Big Assumption. Simply pay attention to any situations that could illustrate that your Big Assumption might not be true.*** Try to identify at least four or five such situations and describe them in the left-hand column of the following chart in your Change Journal. Then, in the right-hand column, write down how you can see or imagine that your Big Assumption might be wrong (or at least not always right).

Counter-Observations Template

Describe the situations where your Big Assumption might possibly be wrong (including your thoughts & feelings).	**How could what happened possibly suggest a way that your Big Assumption is wrong or distorted?**
Counter Observation #1:	Counter Observation #1:
Counter Observation #2:	Counter Observation #2:
Counter Observation #3:	Counter Observation #3:
Counter Observation #4:	Counter Observation #4:

Ron's Counter Observations

Ron conducted his counter observations in the same week that he was observing how his Big Assumption was showing up in all parts of his life and holding him back from his weight-loss goals. At the end of the week, he hadn't written down any situations that seemed to illustrate how his Big Assumption might not be true. But as he thought back, he remembered that – by chance – he had been sick the week before and had not eaten as much as he usually did. The more he thought about that, the more he realized that situation actually was a counter observation he could learn from.

Ron's Big Assumption: I assume no matter what my friends do I'll feel less a part of things and that I am missing out on the full experience if I am not eating like my friends are eating.

Ron's Counter Observations:

Describe the situations where your Big Assumption might possibly be wrong (including your thoughts & feelings).	**How could what happened possibly suggest a way that your Big Assumption is wrong or distorted?**
I had a really bad cold last week. Nothing tasted good, so I just ate much less than I usually do. None of my friends teased me for not eating.	It's really easy to tell people you don't want to eat because you're sick. I actually thought maybe I should get some kind of chronic illness – or tell people that – so that I can lose weight. Just kidding.
So, there are lots of people who don't eat just because other people are. Now that I'm paying attention, I see that they just take less food or say no to something, and it's fine. No big deal. They seem to be having a perfectly good time hanging out with other people without having to eat so much.	Well, once people get used to what you eat and how much, then they just expect that. So if people do get used to me eating less, then it will be much easier. Maybe I can still feel a part of the full experience without eating so much too?

Then he thought about whether there were things that *other* people did that would suggest his own BA might not be true. It didn't take long for him to realize that there were lots of other people he knew who seemed to eat less (or even eat nothing at all) in situations when Ron would feel social pressure to eat. He decided to record something about those situations as well.

Miriam's Counter Observations

At first, Miriam wasn't sure she would be able to do counter observations since she was already trying to change her behavior by eating better and exercising more. But she decided that she could learn quite a bit by paying close attention to what was happening as she tried to make these changes and what she might learn about her Big Assumptions, including the new one she uncovered in last week's observations. She also was surprised to find that there were some situations that were not specifically related to food that might begin to suggest there could be flaws in her Big Assumptions.

Miriam's Big Assumption: I assume if I don't criticize myself harshly, I'll slack off too much.

Miriam's Counter Observations:

Describe the situations where your Big Assumption might possibly be wrong (including your thoughts & feelings).	How could what happened possibly suggest a way that your Big Assumption is wrong or distorted?
Since I've been working long hours, my to-do list of other stuff has been growing longer and longer. There are items that have been on there for weeks. I was feeling really stressed out about it. But I talked myself through it and did a quick prioritization. I gave myself 20 minutes to get the most important ones done, and I did. I felt really good about doing something proactive to relieve my stress. And hey, I didn't even think about eating something during the stress, or to congratulate myself afterwards!!	There's at least one example where I felt stressed and didn't have to eat to feel better. Maybe it helped that it wasn't stress in any relationship?
I woke up today feeling good. I made good eating choices all morning and am feeling positive about them. Now it is almost lunch time and I'm feeling hungry. But I also feel good to be hungry – like it isn't so hard to handle.	When things are calm and not stressful, I feel like I can eat much more reasonably. I can stand to be hungry.
A new yoga instructor taught today's class. She had us do a pose that was new and really hard for me. I practically fell on my face. But I felt determined to try it again.	I realized that I didn't criticize myself harshly for screwing up, and I was able to keep going in class! It helped that this particular teacher gave us a heads up that it would be hard, and I could see that other people were struggling too.

What Have You Learned From Your Self-Observations?

Self-observations often lead people to big insights, including discovering just how costly it has been to be operating as if their Big Assumptions are always 100% accurate; seeing just how thoroughly they have been ignoring information that suggests their Big Assumptions could be wrong; and recognizing their Big Assumptions not only affect their struggles to achieve their health goals, but affect other areas of their lives too (how they do at work, what happens in their intimate relationships, the ways they communicate with their kids, etc.).

Take some time to reread the situations you've described, and the insights you've generated. Answer the following questions in your Change Journal.

Observing the Big Assumption

1. What stands out to you? What do you notice most of all? Any "ah ha" moments?
2. What thoughts, feelings, perspectives, actions, and choices do you experience?
3. Do you see patterns? Are there particular types of people, content areas, circumstances (inside yourself or in the environment) that activate your Big Assumption?

Counter Observations

4. Is the same doubt about your Big Assumption raised across the different instances? Is there anything in common across the examples that might account for the counter-data? (e.g., particular types of people, content areas, circumstances, inside yourself or in the environment).
5. Do you think or feel differently about your Big Assumption now after observing it for a while? If so, describe what has changed.
6. Do you notice any additional Big Assumptions you are making? If so, add these to your 4-column ITC map.

Miriam Takes a Different Perspective on Herself

It was hard for Miriam to look back over all the observations she had made. In her first attempt at the observation exercise, she had trouble even coming up with examples to consider. Some of these situations were very painful to remember, and keeping regular notes and reflections had been hard. She decided that the only way to convince herself to look back at her notes was to imagine that she was reading about someone else, someone she had never even met.

As she began to read, she gasped. "This person sounds so depressed," she realized. "If someone were saying this to me, I would be so upset and worried for her. I would be thinking to myself that no one could possibly be so terrible, and that she is working really hard to convince herself that's true for some reason! I see that every day, I'm constantly criticizing myself and putting myself down. I think it is fine to do this to myself, but I would never think these things were justified if someone else did them!"

The pattern she had been following suddenly looked crystal clear, and she realized that her overeating felt most out of control whenever she was faced with a difficult emotion. "I get stressed, and I eat. I feel sad, and I eat. I feel out of control, and I eat. But here is the thing that is the most unbelievably stupid about that – I am doing this to myself! The more I tell myself I'm an idiot, the more I eat!"

Ron Notices the Pattern He Follows

When Ron looked at his observations, he noticed a clear pattern. He was assuming that he was making other people happy when he ate. He was also assuming that he had no choice but to either make them happy, which he enjoyed doing, or make them unhappy, by eating less or eating healthier. When he had written his map, he had focused mostly on a small group of his closest friends, but the more he observed, the more he could see that he was carrying a more general version of these assumptions around with him wherever we went. He decided to keep track of these more general versions and added them to his map:

- I assume that I am making other people happy when I eat.
- I assume that my only choices are to either make people happy by overeating, or make them unhappy by eating less or eating healthier.

The more he paid attention to others who eat less and eat more healthfully, the more Ron also saw that no one else seemed bothered by those eating habits. No one looked disappointed when these people ate small portions or even turned down a slice of cake. The problem for Ron was that food had been something he really liked a lot and liked to talk about. The way other people talked about their favorite TV shows or swapped stories about their kids was the way Ron interacted with others about good food. "So, I guess I know things could eventually be different for me," Ron explained. "I just think the hardest part will be the beginning – when everyone probably will be expecting me to keep feeding my pie hole and will be just completely confused when I don't. I don't relish all the conversations where my friends will all be saying 'who are you, man?' And I'll be like, 'Yeah. I know, I gotta be somebody else now.'"

We hope that by now you're beginning to appreciate the habit of self-observation. The more conscious you are of what you are doing, why you are doing it, and what happens as a result, the more you can begin to see that your usual ways of thinking and acting are only one choice among many other possibilities. The more you can be on the look-out for situations that can teach you how your thinking might be wrong, the greater the chances that you will change the beliefs that are doing you more harm than good.

That's why we urge you to continue practicing this habit. Moving on to the next chapter? Fine, but keep observing as well. Done with the book? Keep observing. Observing your Big Assumptions helps you to step away from them – and that means taking one small step into the unknown that exists beyond the BA.

Adrian's Counter-Observation

Adrian was an organizational consultant living in Germany. He had been quite overweight ever since he was a boy and had struggled and failed to lose weight for most of his life. Finally, he learned of the ITC approach and drew up his own ITC map. In his Big Assumption column were the following entries:

- I assume that healthy food doesn't taste as good, and will leave me hungry and wanting more.
- I assume that if I don't eat the good stuff (rich, flavorful foods), I will feel unhappy and uncomfortable, never at rest or fully relaxed.
- I assume that eating and drinking are the best ways to forget and recover from anything unpleasant.
- If I don't enjoy life, I will miss what is important.
- If I eat only healthy food, it will cost me too much time.

As an organizational consultant, Adrian often worked with multinational organizations and traveled frequently for his work. Two or three times a year, he would travel to Bangkok for work, usually staying for a few weeks. Each time he returned, he looked forward to eating at his favorite Thai restaurants, where the food was always expertly prepared, colorful and beautifully arranged, and delicious to eat.

One night at dinner, Adrian was appreciating his excellent meal, when he began to look at it more carefully. He noticed that most of what he was eating was actually quite healthy – fresh, crunchy vegetables, whole grain rice, and a light sauce. It was not very salty, or very fatty, but the taste was still quite appealing. With each meal that he ate in Thailand, he noticed that he was enjoying his meal quite a bit *and* that the meals were generally quite healthy and satisfying. After returning from his trip, he weighed himself, which confirmed his impression – he had been eating much more healthily than he typically did, and he had lost a couple of kilos (roughly 5 pounds). Yet he had savored every bite of his food and felt as relaxed and satisfied and happy as he ever did.

Adrian realized that in observing his behavior he had found a naturally-occurring instance that countered his Big Assumption. Without trying to change his behavior, he had simply eaten the way that he always did when he visited Thailand. Yet the typical meal he ate in a Thai restaurant was quite a bit better for him than the meals he ate in most restaurants in other parts of the world. As a result, he had information that contradicted two of his fundamental Big Assumptions:

- I assume that healthy food doesn't taste as good, will leave me hungry and wanting more.
- I assume that if I don't eat the good stuff (rich, flavorful foods), I will feel unhappy and uncomfortable, never at rest or fully relaxed.

"I didn't consciously look to disprove my Big Assumptions," he noted. "And I guess I always rationally knew that healthy food can be tasty. But somewhere in my unconscious I didn't believe that, and when I chose a restaurant or looked at a menu, the richer and fattier foods were always the most appealing. Luckily, that was not the case in Thailand, and that changed everything for me. I suddenly understood how this approach worked, and how it could change not only how I regard food —but all the other areas of my life that I am looking to improve. I felt like I had been duping myself with some, even many, of my beliefs. This was momentarily embarrassing, but long-lastingly liberating!"

6

POP!
Developing Your Picture Of Progress

At first I thought that success would mean that I wouldn't be embarrassed to wear fitted clothes. I thought it would mean others would compliment me on my figure. That was the first stage, and I lost 10-12 kilos. But the more I did this work, the more I learned, and I began to add more and more things to my map. You see, I began to realize that I didn't want to be doing all this work for anybody else. Just myself. I think this took a while to dawn on me and become part of an overall way I was seeing everything differently. Success became about being who I wanted to be – a healthy human in a healthy body. I lost another 12 kilos.

— *Elaine*

Albert Einstein had a great deal of wisdom to share about what it takes to think deeply, solve problems, and discover new territory. We've already passed along his good advice about the importance of really understanding a problem before you try to solve it. Now we're going to borrow another of his commonly quoted observations. Einstein believed that if you really want to achieve something amazing, you have to do some mental work in advance – you need to fully picture what you want to happen, and you have to begin believing that you can pull it all off. And if you can do that mental work, you will be able to reach your goal. In other words, "Imagination is everything. It is the preview of life's coming attractions."

More than half a century after Einstein's death, brain science has proven many of his speculations true. Today, top performers in all kinds of professions such as sports and the arts also know that creating a vivid picture of what it will be like for them to perform at the top of their abilities, and to succeed in their goals, helps them make that dream a reality. They begin to make a new future more real for themselves right now. They begin to develop not only a belief that they can reach their goals, but also to imagine how they will be thinking, acting, and feeling in order to reach their goals.

Doing, Thinking, Feeling: Imagine Your Picture of Progress

Creating a Picture of Progress gives you a structured way to imagine what it will be like to reach your improvement goal by overturning your Big Assumptions. It helps you imagine your new behavior, yes, but also your new thinking and feeling. We are helping you here to create optimistic expectations for what you will be able to achieve. This type of visualization has been shown to help individuals set and reach higher goals of all sorts, helping them also to predict and overcome the obstacles they will face along the way. What you are trying to do is imagine the specific ways you will be making changes and you will be different. Imagine yourself making these changes through persistent, vigilant, and deliberate work.

Creating this picture will show you how the energy you invest in this change process will pay off, and how the changes are likely to show up. If it helps, imagine you are presenting this document as an official report to the research organization that hired you. You are showing how you and people like you will be different once you find out that these Big Assumptions are actually inaccurate.

The template for your POP looks a bit like the one for you immunity map.

Improvement Goal and Big Assumptions	First Noticeable Steps Forward	Significant Progress	Full Success
Write your Column 1 Improvement Goal here, as well as the Big Assumptions that you are focusing on.	Imagine that you have begun to take *First Steps* toward overturning your immunities and reaching your Column 1 improvement goal ***by altering your Big Assumptions***. What are you doing differently? Thinking differently? How are you feeling differently?	Imagine that you have made *Significant Progress* in overturning your immunities and toward reaching your Column 1 improvement goal ***by altering your Big Assumptions.*** What are you doing differently? Thinking differently? How are you feeling differently?	Imagine that you have had *Full Success* in overturning your immunities and reached your Column 1 improvment goal ***by altering your Big Assumptions***. What are you doing differently? Thinking differently? How are you feeling differently?

A thoughtfully completed POP can lead you to insights equally powerful as those that arose in your ITC map. In the following pages, we'll walk you through how to complete a POP step-by-step. But to give you an idea of what you are working toward, we want to show you a completed one. Here is what Ron's completed POP (based on overturning the new Big Assumptions he had found by doing Observations) looked like:

Ron -- Picture of Progress

Improvement Goal and Big Assumptions	First Noticeable Steps Forward	Significant Progress	Full Success
I'm committed to getting better at eating healthier when I'm around other people – at the bar, at parties, at meetings where there is food. I assume that I am making other people happy when I eat. I assume that my only choices are to either make people happy by overeating, or make them unhappy by eating less or eating healthier.	I think about my reasons for eating or drinking something. I think about if I want that thing really or am just doing it because people want me to. I look at people who don't eat or drink as much as I do to see how they can say "no thank you" without making people mad. I make plans to do things with my friends that don't mean we have to eat or drink together. I pay attention to enjoying this different kind of time spent with them. I don't like it when I see how much has to change, how far I have to go, but I try to remember that I am further than I was before and Rome wasn't built in a day. Stay the course. Then I feel recharged.	I tell my friends that I'm trying to lose weight and get healthier. I start to say "no thank you" sometimes to food. I eat more fruit and vegetables. I find out which ones I like and enjoy eating them. I get up early and go running before work. I go to the bar less often but don't mind because I'm doing other things I like by myself or with my friends. I feel good that I am actually doing things that I have wanted to do for a while. I tell myself that what I eat and drink is up to me. If I eat well, good on me. If I overeat or eat junk, there is only myself to blame. You reap what you sow. I don't particularly feel I am missing out, and I don't feel like my buddies think I'm a weirdo.	I eat what I want to eat, not because I think other people want me to eat something or eat more of something. I feel good about making my own choices. I can still feel like a part of things and having a great time even when I eat less than my friends. I don't talk about food all the time. I feel excited about new things in my life. I feel like I am in control. I feel like I can make my own choices. I lose weight and exercise regularly. I feel better – healthier and more energetic. I am not worried that people like based on what I eat or don't eat. They just like me.

What a Picture of Progress is NOT

- A Picture of Progress is *not* intended to be a *plan* for change. It doesn't give you "marching orders" or tell you *how* this progress is going to unfold. Once you create it, you are not then supposed to "execute" it. All this would pull you back into thinking you'll make changes through will power and self-discipline. Again, our approach for creating change is about getting your mind right. The POP helps with this not by consciously and deliberately providing you a road map to follow, but by helping you begin to create new images and neural pathways for the changes to come.

- And we don't want you to daydream and create some lovely fantasy world in which you are thin and beautiful, or pretend that the type of changes you hope to make will happen magically or overnight. This type of daydreaming may lead you to mentally enjoy some idealized future world, but it actually has been shown to *decrease* motivation and investment in what is involved in making those changes. It *does not* help people prepare for upcoming obstacles or setbacks.

- You are also not focusing on (or even including) any hoped for changes that are not within your own control. For example, you should not imagine that your own weight loss will inspire others to lose weight. You should not make plans for how losing weight will suddenly make your boss nicer to you. Someone else might get inspired to change their behavior, but ultimately, that is up to them and is not something you can personally engineer. Similarly, you should not imagine that losing weight will change circumstances around you. We are sorry to be the ones to tell you this, but losing weight will not guarantee you extra money to buy a new, sexy wardrobe. It will not make you less bald. It will not prevent you from getting older. Yeah, we know that's hard to accept.

Our point is that we want you to dream *but not* create an unattainable romantic fantasy. We want you to imagine what could really happen for you — not lose all contact with reality. Specifically, we want you to try and sketch out a picture of what life can be like if you are able to make progress on your improvement goal by overturning your Big Assumptions. With those parameters in mind, feel free to close your eyes and build an image.

NOTE: Some people find this exercise extraordinarily difficult to do because of their Big Assumptions. If I have a Big Assumption "I assume that I will fail again like I have always done before," trying to visualize success will be particularly hard. Give it your best shot! If you are working with a partner, check in with him or her. It can be much easier for someone other than ourselves to imagine what it could feel like to no longer be captive of our personal Big Assumptions. But if you get stuck here and your ITC progress begins to stall, better to skip this exercise (at least for now) and move on to the next chapter. As we have said, some exercises can be done in any order, and people have experienced success with our approach even if they don't necessarily do all of the exercises we recommend.

Full Success

In this exercise you will fill out the left-most and right-most columns of your POP chart in your Change Journal, leaving the intermediate columns for later. So the first step is to copy out your original ITC Column 1 improvement goal and your BAs in the left-most column of your POP.

The first picture we'd like you to develop is your vision of what it would be like to have complete, full success in reaching your Column 1 goal. When we first ask people to visualize their own success, they usually offer some specific details about their goals: they hope to wear a smaller dress size, reach a particular number on the scale, describe how they would like to look in a bathing suit, recite measureable health improvements (e.g., cholesterol numbers, blood pressure, etc.), and/or describe increased physical ability (distance/speed at which they can walk or run, etc.). These concrete details are common to what people are most likely to imagine and we encourage you to pay attention to these aspects of your goals. But, as you may have guessed, we're going to ask you to focus your imagination a bit differently. We want you to imagine what it would be like to change your Big Assumptions.

If you were to alter your Big Assumptions, what kinds of amazing things might you be able to do? What might you be able to believe? How might you think differently than you currently do? What might it feel like to be released from your Big Assumptions? How might it physically feel different to have a healthier, fitter, smaller body? Review your ITC map to remind yourself of your immune system and your Big Assumptions, focusing particularly on the one that feels most powerful to you.

Imagine that you have been completely successful in overturning your immunities and have reached your Column 1 improvement goal by *altering your Big Assumptions.*

Write your answers to the following questions in the "Full Success" section of the Picture of Progress exercise in your Change Journal.

- Imagine what your new **behaviors** are. What are you now able to do? What old behaviors are you able to cut out? (For ideas of what might change, look back at Column 2 of your ITC map.) How do you think you will be able to start doing these things (and stop doing others)?

- Imagine how you might **think** differently when you have fully succeeded. What do you now believe? What are you thinking about? How does the way that you think support the new ways you are able to behave?

- What does it **feel** like to have completely reached your improvement goal? What does it feel like to have changed your Big Assumptions? What does it feel like to be living in a body that you have been able to transform? What does it feel like to be behaving and thinking in new ways?

Give yourself lots of time to generate a detailed picture in your mind and on the page. When you feel like you have a full description, enter these specific ideas into the column that is **farthest to the right.** (We'll come back to the *First Steps Forward* column and the *Significant Progress* columns after completing *Full Success*. Trust us. It's easier this way.)

Ron – Full Success

Here is what Ron came up with when he imagined what he'd be *doing* differently, how he'd be *feeling* differently, and how he'd be *thinking* differently if he overturned his two key Big Assumptions. (I assume that I am making other people happy when I eat. I assume that my only choices are to either make people happy by overeating, or make them unhappy by eating less or eating healthier.):

I eat what I want to eat, not because I think other people want me to eat something or eat more of something. I feel good about making my own choices.

- I can still feel like a part of things and have a great time even when I eat less than my friends.

- I don't talk about food all the time. I feel excited about new things in my life.

- I feel like I am in control. I feel like I can make my own choices.

- I lose weight and exercise regularly. I feel better – healthier and more energetic.
- I am not worried that people like me based on what I eat or don't eat. They just like me.

Miriam – Full Success

Miriam spent quite a long time coming to her version of "Full Success." She found it difficult – and even a little bit scary to try to imagine that she could actually get to a place in her life that was so completely different from where she was now. She spent several days mulling over a "vision" for her success but still felt like she couldn't really imagine anything that felt realistic, like something she could actually do.

But in the meantime, she had begun reading the book *Women, Food, and God* by Geneen Roth and felt like the author was speaking directly to her. As Roth described other women who compulsively overeat to blot out their own feelings of inadequacy, pain, and shame, Miriam felt a shock of recognition. She recognized the fear of her own emotions. She recognized the ways she continually berated herself. She was drawn to the idea of coming to accept herself and her body and the advice to practice meditation and self-compassion.

Finally, she put on some relaxing, spa-like music, closed her eyes, and allowed herself to imagine a new kind of future for herself, one in which she had overturned her Big Assumption that if she didn't criticize herself harshly, she would slack off. After about 15 minutes, she opened her eyes and slowly began to write down the specifics of what she was starting to picture. She returned to her list again later that day to add a few more items. Her final list was:

- My healthy eating and exercise habits are the way I prefer to live. I am happy with my eating habits, my weight and my appearance. I have nothing to prove, nothing to hide and nothing to change. I am not worrying about how others see me. I am good enough as I am!
- I feel good about myself. I value my own opinions. I feel at ease in my own skin. I feel whole. I believe these feelings will fuel my sense of well-being. I'm not worrying about how others see me, and I'm not being self-critical.
- It has been a long but worthwhile journey. I feel much more in control of my actions, emotions and expectations and do not use food to deal with stress, loneliness or sadness. I have found new ways to deal with my stress.

- When I talk to myself, I am usually positive and affirming regarding my abilities to maintain good health and accomplish my goals.
- I feel gratified while I eat because my choices around food are healthy for me. Feeling comfortably full feels great. I eat for fitness and pleasure.
- I feel more confident, more in control, stronger, healthier, more vibrant.
- I'm taking more time to relax.
- Sometimes I eat something that feels like a treat, but when I do that, I don't worry or get mad. I can enjoy it and return to my healthier habits.
- I am happy, satisfied, and full!

First Steps Forward

Now that you have a clear idea of what Full Success might be like for you, it should be easier to imagine the journey from here to there. So we recommend that you imagine what the journey will look like when it has just begun. What might it look like to take some first steps in this journey? What would you be doing differently? How would you be feeling and thinking differently? These steps will take you in the direction of Full Success, but they are first steps, and they will likely involve a bit of work and some new learning, as well as exciting developments that mean you are no longer at the starting gate but are measurably on your way. Think about these entries as things that you feel like you realistically can and want to do right now. We often recommend that people think about adding things like these:

- I tell someone else about what I am working on.
- I find others who have succeeded in working through similar immunities by doing something like reading books on this topic, talking to others I know, or joining a support group.
- I pay attention to the times when I do things that undermine my improvement goal (such as the things I listed in Column 2 of my ITC map).

We offer those ideas to start you thinking, but we want you to come up with a picture that makes sense for your own personal journey. What kinds of new behaviors might be important as you start out? What might you learn first about yourself and your BAs? What will it feel like to begin to see real progress and also see what still lies ahead? What kinds of things would you be able to do now that move you out of the starting gate?

Imagine that you have begun to take First Steps toward overturning your immunities and reaching your Column 1 improvement goal *by altering your Big Assumptions.*

Write your answers to the next set of questions in the "First Steps" section of the Picture of Progress exercise, second from the left, in your Change Journal.

- What are your ***behaviors*** at this point in the process? What have you been trying to do (and trying not to do)? What are you doing that helps you make these changes to your behavior?

- How are you learning to ***think*** differently? Have you begun to question or challenge your Big Assumptions? What are you thinking about? How do you practice thinking that can support the behaviors you are starting to practice?

- What does it ***feel*** like to be taking First Steps Forward, to be behaving and thinking in new ways? What does it feel like to set off on a path to learn about and change your Big Assumptions?

Ron's First Steps Forward

Ron struggled a little to come up with ideas for this stage of his journey. But we emphasized to him it isn't necessary to get everything perfect. He relaxed, and eventually came up with Doing, Thinking, and Feeling entries, imagining what might be different if he could begin to overturn his Big Assumptions. (I assume that I am making other people happy when I eat. I assume that my only choices are to either make people happy by overeating, or make them unhappy by eating less or eating healthier.)

- I think about my reasons for eating or drinking something. I think about if I really want that thing or am just doing it because people want me to.

- I look at people who don't eat or drink as much as I do to see how they can say "no thank you" without making people mad.

- I make plans to do things with my friends that don't mean we have to eat or drink together. I pay attention to enjoying this different kind of time spent with them.

- I don't like it when I see how much has to change, how far I have to go, but I try to remember that I am further than I was before and Rome wasn't built in a day. Stay the course. Then I feel recharged.

Miriam's First Steps Forward

If creating her "Full Success" description was motivating to Miriam, the "First Steps Forward" description was even more inspiring to her. "I can see how it can happen now," she said slowly. "I'm not saying it is going to happen. I'm not quite there yet in terms of my self-belief. But it does feel like there is a way forward for me, and I don't think I've been able to picture that before. I can imagine that I begin to change the way I eat and feel and think if I am no longer criticizing myself so harshly." She wrote:

- I am beginning to follow the techniques I know are necessary to lose weight. I identify new and healthy recipes that I want to make. I regularly walk on the treadmill.

- I pay attention to my body and how I eat. I notice: when do I feel hunger? When, where and how do I eat? When do I feel full?

- I pay more attention to my emotions. What do I feel before, during, after I eat? What leads me to be stressed?

- I keep in mind that part of me will feel hopeful and optimistic while another part of me will feel scared, that it is hard to take the first step. That's OK.

- I pay attention to the negative messages that I send to myself.

- I pay attention to how I respond to others' criticisms of me.

- I schedule a set time to meditate or listen to my stress management CD (e.g., right after lunch).

- I finish reading Geneen Roth's book.

Significant Progress

By now you are probably getting the hang of this exercise, and you can most likely tackle the last "imagining" without much further prompting from us. You know what just getting started might look and feel like. You know what complete success might look like and feel like. What will this place in the middle (Significant Progress) be like for you?

Imagine that you have made Significant Progress in overturning your immunities and toward reaching your Column 1 improvement goal by altering your Big Assumptions. You're not just starting, but you're not fully there yet either.

Write your answers in the "Significant Progress" section of the Picture of Progress exercise in your Change Journal.

- What ***behaviors*** have you adopted at this point in the process? What are you now able to do? What old behaviors are you able to cut out? What are you doing that helps you make these changes to your behavior?

- What kind of progress have you made in ***thinking*** differently? What do you now believe? What are you thinking about? How do you practice thinking that can support the new ways you are able to behave?

- What does it ***feel*** like to be making Significant Progress (but not yet reaching Full Success)? How might you have changed your Big Assumptions? How do you keep those Big Assumptions from feeling like they are 100% true? What does it feel like to be behaving and thinking in new ways? What does it feel like to be transforming your body?

Ron – Significant Progress

Ron looked back at his improvement goal, his first steps, and his picture of full success. It was starting to seem almost logical to imagine the intermediate steps that would bring him to his goal. He wrote down how it would look when he had made "Significant Progress" in overturning his BAs. (I assume that I am making other people happy when I eat. I assume that my only choices are to either make people happy by overeating, or make them unhappy by eating less or eating healthier.)

- I tell my friends that I'm trying to lose weight and get healthier.
- I start to say "no thank you" sometimes to food.
- I eat more fruit and vegetables. I find out which ones I like and enjoy eating them.
- I get up early and go running before work.
- I go to the bar less often but don't mind because I'm doing other things I like by myself or with my friends.

Then he asked himself how he would be *feeling* differently and thinking differently in order to be doing these things. He added:

- I feel good that I am actually doing things that I have wanted to do for a while.
- I tell myself that what I eat and drink is up to me. If I eat well, good on me. And I enjoy what I eat. If I overeat or eat junk, there is only myself to blame. You reap what you sow.
- I don't particularly feel I am missing out, and I don't feel like my buddies think I'm a weirdo.

Miriam – Significant Progress

When Miriam started to think about "Significant Progress," she was surprised to find her ideas came more quickly. While it had been difficult to create a vision of what might truly feel like "Full Success" that *also* felt believable and achievable, that hard work was helping her now. "I started allowing myself to believe that criticizing myself wasn't actually helping me, and that I have even the tiniest chances of meeting my goals. Thinking about what that would look like to be working toward that only gave me more hope and more belief!" she stated. "And while it still felt scary to write my ideas down – which makes them feel even more real – it also gives me so much motivation about what is really possible for me." Here is her list:

- Every day, I am walking on the treadmill or doing yoga for at least 30 minutes. I am following Weight Watchers' guidelines. I make time to prepare and eat a healthy dinner of meat and veggies. I drink at least 5 glasses of water and remember to take supplements daily.

- It doesn't feel as hard now to 'diet' as the healthy behaviors are part of my routine. I honestly believe that I can reach my weight loss goals and maintain a healthy lifestyle. I am noticeably lighter/thinner and feel the benefits in how I move and how my clothes fit. Temptations are easier to avoid. And WOW, it feels good when people notice!

- I am better able to identify what types of situations will cause strong emotional reactions for me — the kind that could lead me to want to eat —and plan for how to handle them. When I can identify these situations ahead of time, I prepare for them — by making sure I have healthy food, by tuning in to my emotions, by practicing meditation, etc. I tell myself I can handle my emotions in new ways, and keep track of what works.

- When I start to criticize myself and get negative, I notice and interrupt myself. I think of at least one more positive message I can tell to myself instead. I stop myself whenever I start to engage in self-punishment or self-criticism. I am worrying less about what others think of me.

- When I want to eat, I ask myself why I am eating – because I am hungry or because I feel stressed, sad, angry, etc. If I am hungry I eat. If I have an emotional need, I have developed strategies for how to help myself feel better.

- I forgive myself when I make mistakes. When I mess up, I focus on improving my actions at the next meal.

- I am losing weight and enjoy the satisfaction this brings when I get on the scale.

Miriam -- Picture of Progress

Improvement Goal and Big Assumptions	First Noticeable Steps Forward	Significant Progress	Full Success
→	→	→	
I'm committed to getting better at creating and following new lifelong food habits – no fad diets, no drastic approaches that I can't keep up. I assume if I don't criticize myself really harshly, I'll slack off too much.	I am beginning to follow the techniques I know are necessary to lose weight. I identify new and healthy recipes that I want to make. I regularly walk on the treadmill. I pay attention to my body and how I eat. I notice: when do I feel hunger? When, where and how do I eat? When do I feel full? I pay more attention to my emotions. What do I feel before, during, after I eat? What leads me to be stressed? I keep in mind that part of me will feel hopeful and optimistic while part of me will feel scared, that it is hard to take the first step. And that's OK. I pay attention to the negative messages that I send to myself. I pay attention to how I respond to others' criticisms of me.	Every day, I am walking on the treadmill or doing yoga for at least 30 minutes. I am following Weight Watchers' guidelines. I make time to prepare and eat a healthy dinner of meat and veggies. I drink at least 5 glasses of water and remember to take supplements daily. It doesn't feel as hard now to 'diet' as the healthy behaviors are part of my routine. I honestly believe that I can reach my weight loss goals and maintain a healthy lifestyle. I am noticeably lighter/thinner and feel the benefits in how I move and how my clothes fit. Temptations are easier to avoid. And WOW, it feels good when people notice! I am better able to identify what types of situations will cause strong emotional reactions for me – the kind that could lead me to want to eat – and plan for how to handle them.	My healthy eating and exercise habits are the way I prefer to live. I am happy with my eating habits, my weight and my appearance. I have nothing to prove, nothing to hide and nothing to change. I am not worrying about how others see me. I am good enough as I am! I feel good about myself. I value my own opinions. I feel at ease in my own skin. I feel whole. I believe these feelings will fuel my sense of well-being. I'm not worrying about how others see me, and I'm not being self-critical. It has been a long but worthwhile journey. I feel much more in control of my actions, emotions and expectations and do not use food to deal with stress, loneliness or sadness. I have found new ways to deal with my stress.

Miriam -- Picture of Progress Continued

Improvement Goal and Big Assumptions →	First Noticeable Steps Forward →	Significant Progress →	Full Success
	I schedule a set time to meditate or listen to my stress management CD (e.g., right after lunch). I read Geneen Roth's book.	When I can identify these situations ahead of time, I prepare for them — by making sure I have healthy food, by tuning in to my emotions, by practicing meditation, etc. I tell myself I can handle my emotions in new ways, and keep track of what works. When I start to criticize myself and get negative, I notice and interrupt myself. I think of at least one more positive message I can tell to myself instead. I stop myself whenever I start to engage in self-punishment or self-criticism. I am worrying less about what others think of me. When I want to eat, I ask myself why I am eating – because I am hungry or because I feel stressed, sad, angry, etc. If I am hungry I eat. If I have an emotional need, I have developed strategies for how to help myself feel better. I forgive myself when I make mistakes. When I mess up, I focus on improving my actions at the next meal. I am losing weight and enjoy the satisfaction this brings when I get on the scale.	When I talk to myself, I am usually positive and affirming regarding my abilities to maintain good health and accomplish my goals. I feel gratified while I eat because my choices around food are healthy for me. Feeling comfortably full feels great. I eat for fitness and pleasure. I feel more confident, more in control, stronger, healthier, more vibrant. I'm taking more time to relax. Sometimes I eat something that feels like a treat, but when I do that, I don't worry or get mad. I can enjoy it and return to my healthier habits. I am happy, satisfied, and full!

How's Your Picture of Progress Coming Along?

Make sure your Picture of Progress is a picture of how your change will look and feel; not how you make these changes, how others will change, the world will change, or how change will happen by luck or chance. While we may hope that other changes will happen as we change ourselves, ultimately, we can't control those things.

Look at what you wrote in each column and compare it with what you have in the other columns. For example, after thinking about what your "First Steps" might look like you might have new ideas for what will be "Significant Progress" and "Full Success." If, for instance, you wrote in "First Steps" that you would stop eating your lunch at restaurants so as to avoid the temptation of ordering and eating more than you want to, consider what you will be able to do when you are further along. Maybe when you have made "Significant Progress" you will have identified a handful of restaurants that offer at least some healthy foods and smaller servings, and you are able to go out to eat at least once a week without sabotaging your progress. You still need to work hard to make sure you don't order some of your old favorites. And then at "Full Success" you might enjoy going to restaurants for lunch because you don't find those "old favorites" appealing. You know how to choose foods wherever you go that are healthy and delicious, and you don't feel scared that you'll end up sabotaging your progress.

If you are having a hard time with this exercise, read through the examples we have provided to see if they help clarify what we are asking you to do, and if they might give you some ideas for what could be in your Picture of Progress.

Remind yourself that the purpose of identifying these progress steps is *not* to begin immediately trying to accomplish them. They are not rungs on a ladder you should now start to climb. The whole point of the *immune system* concept is that change is *not* a straight-forward matter as people often think. Instead, we hope that working through this exercise has provided you with a sense of direction, with energy and optimism, with a clear idea of what you will need to learn to do, and with a realistic idea of the pace of improvement. Some people experience their POP as a game-changer (something "pops" for them mentally or emotionally) but others do not, and it's fine either way. These "pops" occur (when and if they do) during these exercises because you are working here on getting your *mind right* to get your *weight right*. Getting to lasting change, looked at from the outside, seems to be about small, incremental steps, taken over time, with success building upon success. But to produce this arc on the outside requires a less linear set of changes on the inside to your Big Assumptions.

Your Picture of Progress also shows you what kinds of changes you will make internally. For example, imagine that your Column 1 improvement goal is to eat a healthy, vegetarian diet, and *your Big Assumption is that eating such a diet will cause others to judge you, pressure you, or think you are judging them.* Creating your Picture of Progress guides you to imagine what you will do, think, and feel that will help you tune out others' expectations and reactions. That doesn't tell you how this is going to happen, but it begins to prepare your mind *for* it to happen.

As is the case with your ITC map, you may find that your ideas about future success will change as you learn more from the other exercises to follow, and as you actually begin to make more progress. For that reason, it may be useful to periodically review and revise your Picture of Progress as you discover new thoughts and feelings along your way. Finally, your Picture of Progress will be a useful way to check in at the end of this book (and thereafter) to gauge what progress you have actually made and where you are on the journey, not just to getting your weight right but your mind right as well.

Eleanor's Picture of Progress

Eleanor's improvement goal is not to lose weight. She has already done that, as she has before. Her goal is to get better at *keeping it off.* She chose to focus on two of the many Big Assumptions she uncovered in her immunity map:

- I assume that keeping off the weight will be hard because I won't have the rewards of seeing the number on the scale go down.
- I assume that continuing to eat less will start to feel very "blah."

When she began drafting her Picture of Progress, she tried hard to imagine what it would be like to no longer hold these beliefs. After thinking for a while, she came up with one idea of what would constitute "Full Success" – a way she could continue to reward herself, without seeing changing numbers on a scale, a way to not feel the "blahs":

- I will enjoy being able to buy new clothes each season as styles change. I have always wanted to be trendy, but the styles never looked good on me.

Once she started thinking about indulgences, lots of new ideas came quickly to her:

- I will start taking classes toward becoming a certified masseuse – regularly giving and getting massages as a way to relax, indulge myself, and manage my stress.
- When my lease is up, I will move closer to the park so that I can enjoy taking walks and being out in nature.
- I will schedule my aerobics classes on weekday evenings, so that the exercise allows me to release my stress from the day.

As she wrote, Eleanor was surprised to see how many of her ideas would not have to wait until she reached "Full Success" but were changes she could begin working on immediately. "I got really excited," she gushed, "because since losing weight, I have felt like I missed having a goal and watching my progress. That's why I was so worried I would gain it back again. But now I feel like I have lots of new plans and goals that include ways for me to keep the weight off!"

7

Charting The Biography Of Your Big Assumptions*

I knew my Big Assumptions were connected to my past. I have very addictive behavior that shows up in how I eat. But they have shown up in every other area of my life too. I can be very needy, very co-dependent. I am always asking for attention. I knew I needed to figure out where these things came from. I began to find out why I always felt unhappy with my work, my marriage and my family. ITC helped me recognize what I was doing and generate new distance from my assumptions. I have a new relationship to food and a new understanding of my relationships.

— *Ulrich*

Biography – Approach #1

We're going to ask you to jump into this exercise without providing you with much upfront explanation. Just play with us here, and you'll see where this exercise gets you after you do it. We think that when people jump into the exercise without thinking much about what they are trying to uncover or learn, their experience tends to be more powerful. This happens because they uncover things they never would have unearthed if they hadn't approached the exercise with a very open mind, free of expectation. Ready to try it yourself?

---

* We want to acknowledge an organization we admire, Learning as Leadership (www.learnaslead.org). This exercise is an only slightly modified, ITC-oriented, version of their original creation.

If you cast back in memory over the first 15 or 16 years of your life, and are asked to capture a handful of negatively-tinged experiences, what comes to mind?

See if you can identify five or six memories that were disturbing, embarrassing, upsetting, infuriating, or scary, for example. They don't have to be events that were momentous; it may even be better if they are not. They may even seem like tiny, mundane, common early-life experiences, the sorts of things that now seem like the normal bumps and bruises of growing up. Nonetheless, they stick with you because these are what came to mind. Record these events in Column 1 of the Biography table found in your Change Journal (p. 18).

Events (the headlines)	What I was thinking at that time	What I was feeling at that time	Lessons learned/ conclusions drawn at that time

Once you have listed the headlines of these events "vertically" in Column 1, start with the first headline and work "horizontally" across Columns 2-4. Column 4 is asking what you think you (as a child who was 4 or 7 or 13) concluded at the time about yourself or "the world," adults, or your parents, in particular. What lessons did you take away then from those experiences? Then work across the columns for each of your memories until the whole table is filled in.

When your biography chart is complete, look at the collection of lessons learned in Column 4 to see if there are any connections you can make between them and your Big Assumptions in Column 4 from your immunity map.

What connections, if any, do you make between the fourth column on your Biography Chart and the fourth column on your ITC map?

Write your answers in the space provided after the Biography table in your Change Journal. If you want to see an example first, read on to see Ron's biography table and his further reflections.

Ron—Biography Approach #1

Events (the headlines)	What I was thinking at that time	What I was feeling at that time	Lessons learned/ conclusions drawn at that time
Big family meals as a kid – every Sunday, every holiday. Everybody ate a lot, and you were always told to eat more.	If I eat, people like that.	If I eat, people seem happy. That's good. I feel connected to my family.	People want you to eat. They want you to like their food and to eat a lot of it. That makes them feel good, and then they like to tell everybody how much you ate. Like they were proud of me. I learned to feel good at making them happy this way.
In high school, all my friends were on the football team. One guy stopped playing because he wasn't really big enough or good enough to play much. After he quit, we didn't really hang out with him so much anymore.	He isn't like us. It is OK to be different but then you might not have the same friends.	Glad I'm still on the team.	People really like you to be like them. Your friends are your friends because you have things in common.
In my 20s, I started to drink a lot. I ate a lot too, but I never gained weight. My girlfriend always said how lucky I was. She would always say, "I wish I could eat like that, but I'd look like a whale."	Guys are lucky – we can eat whatever we want usually.	I like to do what I want without having to worry about being fat. She always seemed kind of sad and annoyed not to eat what she wanted. I always told her to eat more, but I admit I didn't really want her to be fat. I don't think I really believed that would happen to me too. I wish I still could be like that.	Some people are lucky. Guys are lucky because they don't have to diet. Dieting is not fun and other people will feel sorry for you.

When Ron looked at the situations in his Biography and considered them all together, he quickly saw the connection between his lessons learned and two of his Big Assumptions—that he'll feel less a part of things if he isn't eating like his friends, and that he makes other people happy when he eats. His big insight from reflecting on these long ago events is how much he tied making people happy by eating with feeling included and a part of things. He also felt a twinge of remorse. "I liked being that guy," he mused. "I really enjoyed being able to eat a lot and not worry and the way that people always kind of envied me for that. And I guess I feel like I would still be that guy if I could. The thing is, I can't. I wish I could. But I can't. It's time to grow up."

Once he looked clearly at his BAs compared with the evidence of his adult life, he realized that he had already begun to chart his course toward a healthier existence. He could now begin to move beyond being controlled by his BAs.

As you have seen, this Biography exercise invites you to look back to get some clues where your Big Assumptions came from, and to see how long-standing are their origins. Our Big Assumptions, typically, have been living with us for a while (sometimes for a very long while), and have become part of our skin without our realizing it. Many of the people we work with can trace their Big Assumptions back to the time when they were children, trying to find their places in and make sense of their roles in their families. The exercise helps us locate pivotal experiences, which may or may not have anything to do with food or eating habits, but which contributed to the formation of our Big Assumptions (which *do* have implications for our relationship to food). They may have been formed without our realizing it, when we were quite little, or teens, or adults. They may have been formed in our homes, at school, or at work. As you think back over your own life, see if you can further identify the types of situations, people, events, or contexts that may have led you to develop your Big Assumption in the first place. Then see if you can identify other experiences in your life that also led you to form or believe in your Big Assumption.

Let's take the example of a man named Gabriel who had identified two Big Assumptions: "If I don't eat as much as I can at a meal, I will feel hungry, deprived, and suffer later," and, "if I am deprived of food, I am also deprived of love." When Gabriel was ten his father changed careers, and for a while, the family had little money. For periods of time, the family ate only the least expensive foods – rice, beans, pasta, and potatoes. For special occasions, the family would go out for a meal at a fast food restaurant. During this time, Gabriel's parents were under a great deal of pressure, and Gabriel remembers that they fought a lot, worked constantly, and rarely were able to relax and enjoy themselves. "I remember feeling like the only times we all were together was when we were eating. And when there was enough food, you made sure to eat as much as you could because who knows what would be available later? And I guess I also felt like when we had the least money (and the least food) was when things were the worst – fighting, stress, misery. I must have begun to associate food with love then. Even now, I love it when my wife spends the day in the kitchen cooking a big holiday meal, and we all sit down to eat together. I love those times, and I hate the idea of giving them up. But according to my doctor, things are going to have to change, or I won't even be around to enjoy my family."

Charting the Biography of your Big Assumption can be helpful to your progress in a few important ways. First, we often have a much clearer understanding of why we have been holding this Big Assumption in the first place. Many clients have been looking at their Big Assumptions and seeing them only as the things that are in their way, holding them back from their goals. They look at their Big Assumptions and feel frustrated and annoyed by them. If that's the case for you, exploring the biography of the BA can help you to be a little more forgiving or compassionate toward yourself. There are usually very good reasons why we have developed our BAs. They may have helped us survive in situations that were unsafe. They may even have helped us to succeed in certain ways.

The biography can also be very useful in providing you with a clear set of situations to compare and contrast with your current life. Are the reasons why you developed your Big Assumption still relevant to your life now? As an adult, Gabriel knew that his own family was actually economically comfortable. He had no need to worry about having food to feed his family in the ways that his father had when Gabriel was a boy. So even though his Big Assumptions still felt very real to Gabriel, he knew they were not very relevant to his current life. In understanding how and why our Big Assumptions came to be, we may begin, often without even intending to or realizing it, to change our relationship to them.

Biography – Approach #2

We want to offer you a second, more direct approach to exploring your Big Assumptions. Start by thinking straightforwardly about events or situations in your life that may have helped to create, shape, and support each of your Big Assumptions. Start at the beginning – your earliest memories of your Big Assumption – and trace its course through your life.

What is the "history" of your Big Assumption? When was it born? Are there specific situations, feelings, important events or moments you can recall? How long has your BA been around? What were some of its critical turning points?

Perhaps there is one story, event, snapshot, or episode that captures something from your past that may have gotten your Big Assumption started or served to emphasize its importance. ***Again, do not intentionally change anything you do or think relative to your Big Assumption.*** Enter your answers in your Change Journal.

Some of our clients choose one of these approaches over the other in charting their biographies. Some complete both approaches and find one more intriguing than the other. And some find that each approach provides them with unique insights that complement each other. Recording and reflecting on all the incidents in both approaches can help you fill out your biography so that it includes all the key events and situations. Putting your two biographies together should help you tell the whole story.

What Have You Learned from The Biography of Your Big Assumptions, Approach #2?

Once you have completed the Biography exercises, take some time to look back at the situations you've described, and the insights you've generated.

1. In what ways does the biography explain your Big Assumption? Does it show you any additional Big Assumptions you might be making?

2. To what extent do you feel that the conditions that led you to develop your Big Assumption are
3. relevant to your current life?

Write your answers in the space provided in your Change Journal. If you want to see an example first, read on to see Miriam's biography and her further reflections.

Miriam's—Biography Approach #2

My Big Assumption: I assume if I don't criticize myself really harshly, I'll slack off too much.

My parents were both extremely hard-working, and they expected the same from us kids. I felt like the messages they sent us were always about how important it is to work as hard as you can, that if you stop to celebrate or enjoy what you have done, you will fall behind. In my mind, if you felt good about yourself it meant you were too lazy and too self-indulgent to see that you needed to be working even harder than you were.

When I was in Kindergarten, some of my friends were selected to be in a gifted program at school. I wasn't, and I remember feeling like I must not be smart enough or good enough. I felt like there was something wrong with me, and I was embarrassed. I was always comparing myself with other people and finding ways that they were better than me – thinner, smarter, prettier, more talented.

My parents – my father in particular, and maybe all the men in my family – had very specific ideas about what the girls in the family should be like. We should be thin, pretty, and polite. We should marry in our twenties and then start to have children. We could work, but we should never let our work interfere with our families. My mom always worked, and I think my parents hoped that we wouldn't have to feel the financial pressure they did. But I didn't know what I wanted for myself.

I've been doing what they have wanted for me. I'm married, and I have a family. But I know that they (and Paul) think I take my work too seriously. Part of me wonders why I always feel dissatisfied. Will I never be happy with myself? Will I always be looking for more? Why can't I feel good about what I have? My parents worked so hard and wanted this life for me so much. Paul tells me, "You don't realize how lucky you are. You have all day to be at home with the kids."

Miriam reflected on her own biography and saw that it helped her understand why she had always assumed that something was wrong with her. "Writing this biography has made me realize that I learned that I shouldn't think of myself as special or successful or smart," she commented. "It is hard for me to feel proud of what I have. Better to be constantly looking for how I'm not good enough. It is also hard for me to feel like I deserve more than what I have. Even when I write that down, it feels selfish and also really scary – like wanting it and saying so mean it will be taken away. It is easier to hide and not get too ambitious about anything because I might start to relax and slack off. Then, before you know it, something bad will happen. Or, if I succeed, that would be bad too. I'd be selfish and greedy. I'd see all of the bigger things that are wrong with me. I wouldn't be able to be the kind of daughter my family wants or the wife and mother Paul wants me to be. So, I hide to make other people happy. I hide so that I don't bother them with my own needs."

But Miriam could also see that this message contrasted with the feedback she had been getting at work – that she was a valuable asset to the organization and that she had potential to move up to take on greater responsibility. "I have been brushing off that feedback, telling myself not to take it seriously… and also feeling like I shouldn't take it seriously because I can't fit more work into my schedule. But even if I don't move up in the organization, that doesn't mean I can't take pride in what I am doing!"

Completing the Biography of the Big Assumption finishes the first phase of work you have been doing to overturn your immunities. This phase has been focused on studying your Big Assumptions in particular ways—to see where they came from, how they shape your life now, the costs you bear when they hold you back—and to imagine a future when you will be free from them. All of these different ways of seeing, thinking, wondering, questioning, and interpreting allow us to practice one central skill. Instead of going about your life treating your Big Assumption as if it is part of you, as it has been in the past, you can now hold your Big Assumptions out away from you. You can look *at* them (rather than *through* them), turning them around to see them from different angles, maybe even poking or prodding at them to see what happens to them. We can learn a lot from that kind of study of our BAs, as we also learn how to hold them separately from ourselves. That's hard work! And all that heavy lifting has now gotten us into good shape for the next step: Designing and Running Tests of Your Big Assumptions.

Mariana's Biography – Approach #2

When Mariana created her immunity map, she realized that the fears that kept her from losing weight centered on not wanting to rely on or depend on others. "I'm a single mom of two kids, and I have worked hard to be very independent – of my parents, my former husband, everyone. But I realize that if I'm going to change my lifestyle dramatically, I'm going to need others' help," she wrote. "I'm going to have to ask them for help. I'll need to ask my parents if they can help out with childcare while I go to the gym. I'll need support from my boyfriend so that I'm eating healthier meals." Turning that into her hidden commitment, she wrote, "I'm committed to not feeling like I need anyone for anything." It was very painful for Mariana to admit that she needed help from others. That led her to name one of her Big Assumptions: "I assume if I do need others, and I depend on them, I will be at their mercy. I will feel dependent, weak, and immature."

This Big Assumption was clearly rooted in her own biography:

When I was 18, I made some really dumb decisions. I was fighting a lot with my parents. I hated school. So when I got pregnant, I decided to quit school, get married, and start working. I thought I would be free of others' rules and would be able to make all my own decisions.

But the opposite happened. Without a high school diploma, of course I couldn't find a good job. We had no money, and I knew that we wouldn't be able to raise a baby on what we had. So my parents helped us out. They let us live with them, on the condition that I finish high school. I know that we would never have made it otherwise, but I hated living at home again. I hated going back to school. I was miserable. All I could see was that I was having to live by everyone else's rules for me, and it felt like I was walking around wearing handcuffs and a leash. Everybody wanted me to do what they wanted, and as soon as our son was born, I felt even more trapped.

It took about three years for us to finally move out of my parents' house and to get our own place. But that's when we had our second son, and money got really tight again. My mom was watching our kids so I could take more classes at night to get trained in hotel and hospitality management to make better money. When I was able to make a decent living, I didn't even want to be married anymore. I didn't want to compromise my independence for anyone. We got a divorce.

Over the years, after having two kids and with a career that keeps me around food a lot, I have gained a lot of weight. My boyfriend doesn't really care, but I can't stand how I look and feel. I have tried to lose weight, but I really haven't gotten very far. I know I need to build in more time for exercise, and I know I need to make some big changes in what type of food I buy and how I cook. And I hate to say it, but I don't think I can do that all without some help from others – namely, my parents and my boyfriend. I'm not really worried that they won't help me. But I feel like I have worked so hard to stand on my own feet and make my own choices – to live the way I want to. It just feels terrible to admit that I still depend on other people to help me. I feel like a teenager again. I feel like I never get to be a grown up.

PART THREE

Crossing Over

In these next three chapters, we will teach you how to design, carry out, and debrief a series of experiments that "test" the Big Assumption. For most people, testing their Big Assumptions is the most powerful set of exercises in overturning their immunities, moving beyond them, and accomplishing their goal. If you have followed our advice to hold off on changing your behavior (e.g., eating less or differently, exercising more, joining a gym, having a difficult conversation with a family member), now is the time get ready to go out and *do* something different.

The most important thing to keep in mind is that you are not planning to change your behavior just to see if you can. It is easy to fall back into the stance that changing your behavior is how to accomplish your goal. So remember how our approach is different. By testing key Big Assumptions, you will be *intentionally* changing your behaviors and with a clear purpose in mind: *to learn about the accuracy of your Big Assumption.* In other words, the purpose of designing and running a test is to *get information, not* immediately to improve or *get better.*

As you did earlier, think of yourself as a researcher/explorer trying to make sense of these experiments and forays toward your future, so you can apply what you learn as you move beyond the Big Assumptions that have been holding you back.

8

DESIGNING TESTS

I used to start a new exercise program and tell myself "I'm going to do this." And I would do it for a while, but when I would start to slip I'd say "I'm done with that." I assumed it was an all-or-none thing. Now, there are times when I slip, but I know I can get back to it because I've done it before. I know it's not an all-or-none thing. Also, I used to think that I wasn't going to be able to find time to exercise like I should, but now I know there are ways to find time to exercise without causing problems in other areas of my life. I used to say "forget it, it's not going to happen," and now I try to take advantage of opportunities where I can exercise. I'm exercising more now than ever. I look at exercise from a whole different standpoint now.

— *Scott*

Everything you have been doing up until now has put you in a position to design, run, and make sense of the exercises that will test your Big Assumptions. If your tests raise questions about the validity of your BAs, you will be able to revisit and reconsider your BAs, and eventually even overturn them.

Expect to run multiple tests. It is rare that any Big Assumption can be sufficiently explored and either confirmed, revised, or overturned after running just one or two. Your first tests are deliberately quite safe and modest, and then each successive test grows more ambitious and provides new possibilities for learning.

What is a Test? Why Are We Running Them?

Tests of your Big Assumptions basically involve doing things differently than you would normally do ***to get important information about your Big Assumptions (not to take one step closer to your goal)***. When we design and run a test, we are acting as if our BAs might not be true. We are imagining the possibility that they are not as absolutely true as we have previously felt them to be. For example, if I have been certain that I will feel less happy and more confined if I limit my eating to "proper portions," I will continue quite intelligently, reasonably, and faithfully to overeat and undermine my sincere and urgent goal to lose weight. To test this BA, I might set out to eat proper portions for a week to learn "did I, in fact, feel confined and controlled, as my Big Assumption tells me I must?" I am acting as if my Big Assumption might not be true to see what happens. What happens will help me see whether I should continue to hold my Big Assumption in exactly the same form. Changing my Big Assumption, even a little, can permit big changes in my "immune system."

Notice that we didn't say that I would be eating proper portions *in order to lose a couple pounds*. I may, or may not, lose a couple pounds if I run that test, but that is not the purpose of a test. ***The purpose of a test is to see what happens when you intentionally alter your usual behavior in order to learn about the accuracy of your Big Assumption.***

We cannot emphasize this enough: The purpose of a test is to get *information*, not immediately to improve or get better. It is so easy to focus on whether you can successfully change your behavior and consistently eat proper portions, and whether eating proper portions leads you to lose weight. These are not unimportant. But you didn't need this book to try to bring about change this way. That approach is something you already know how to do. This book is teaching you a whole new approach for you to try to see what results it brings. As we've been saying throughout the book, unless you learn more about the beliefs that got you into your current situation, you will be unable to sustain changes in your behavior.

You already know how to make temporary changes. Any diet will help you lose weight…temporarily. ***Our goal in running tests is to see whether you can disprove the Big Assumptions that have been getting in the way of the changes that will help you stay healthy for a lifetime.***

Planning Your Tests

Every test must be directly connected to one of your Big Assumptions. (Some tests will connect to more than one, but don't try to include more than two.) The Big Assumption you choose should feel like one that has a strong hold on you and that if changed would make a big difference. If you have been actively taking part in the prior exercises, you likely know exactly which Big Assumption you want to test. Something we haven't yet discussed, however, is that your Big Assumption needs to be one that can be *safely* tested. This part is really important, so let's consider a couple of examples.

Let's say your Big Assumption is "If I were to fail to lose weight and keep it off again, then I would not be able to face myself." Designing a test of this Big Assumption as it is currently framed would mean that you would have to fail in order to see if you actually could or couldn't face yourself. Clearly, this test is not safe to run. We are quite happy to say (and would guess you are too!) that we hope you'll *never* find out what you'll do if you lose weight and fail to keep it off again.

In a case like this, you can unpack the Big Assumption a bit, to see if there are other assumptions within it or related to it. For example, imagine the Big Assumption worded somewhat differently: "I cannot tolerate *any* more failure when it comes to my weight." While it may be possible to design a safer test of this assumption, it is still not clear how helpful it would be. Think more about your original Big Assumption and focus on what seems most powerful there – is it the fear of failing? That might lead you to reconsider your assumptions about how failure happens. You may be assuming something like, "If I slip up and am not very strictly keeping to my diet for a day or two, that proves that I will fail again. I assume that in making changes to lose weight I must have an all-or-nothing mentality." Or, it may be the consequence element of the assumption that is most important to explore: "I assume if I slip up *then my family will lose all respect for me*." It's important to unpack these assumptions because whichever one you decide to explore will lead to very different tests.

Here is another example. One of the fears that arose for Clara when she was making her ITC map was that any attempts she made to end her addiction to overeating would lead her to resume other addictive behaviors such as binge drinking, drug use, or cigarette smoking. This led her to the following Big Assumption: "I assume that if I do replace my food addiction with another, even more destructive addiction, I will end up killing myself." OK, as it is written, that assumption is clearly not testable. But by now, you can probably begin to identify other, related assumptions that Clara could test. Here are a few possibilities we see:

- I assume that if I work to end one addiction, I will necessarily replace it with another.
- I assume that I cannot successfully treat the underlying cause of my addictive behaviors.
- I assume that I cannot take good care of myself – physically or psychologically.
- I assume that I cannot take control of my life.

You can probably identify several more possibilities for Clara. In fact, we find it is almost always easier to see the assumptions other people are making than it is to see our own. So if you are having trouble identifying a Big Assumption of yours that is safe enough to test, ask your partner if you are working with one. Otherwise, it might be a good idea to ask a trusted friend or colleague for help.

As you're choosing which Big Assumption to test, keep these suggestions in mind:

Be sure that the assumption you have chosen is one that feels ***quite powerful to you***. Ask yourself which BA jumps out at you as the one that most gets in your way. Or, imagine that you can change any single Big Assumption in your map. Which one would make the biggest, most positive difference for you?

The Big Assumption you choose must be **safely *testable.*** Can you imagine some kind of information or data that would help you see that this BA is not true? Is yours so catastrophic that you could never test it? Hint: a BA with words like *die, be fired, or have a nervous breakdown* isn't ready to be tested yet. However, there may be other assumptions that are part of that BA that are safer to test.

If your BA is too extreme to test, try reworking it so that testing it will be a safer, more informative exercise. For example, if your BA says, "I assume if I lose the weight my wife will go into a deep depression," you could change it to the more testable "I assume my losing weight would be threatening and disturbing to my wife." You could test this by *asking* her!

Designing Your First Test

Once you have chosen which Big Assumption to test, write it down in the left hand column in the template in your Change Journal. The next step is to design your first experiment to challenge it.

Question 1: What Big Assumption are you going to test? Add it to the first column.

My Big Assumption Says:	So I will (Change my Behavior This Way)...	And collect the following data ...	In Order to Find Out Whether ...

When you plan a test, it makes sense to think first about what could happen that could disprove your Big Assumptions. To illustrate, let's imagine how a client named Patricia could test one of her BAs: ***I will feel less happy and more confined if I limit my eating to "proper portions."*** Patricia's goal for designing a test is to imagine the possibility that she might find out she will *not* feel less happy and will *not* feel confined by eating proper portions. Her next step is to imagine a test she could design that might lead to that revelation. What could she do? Well, an obvious answer would be: she could simply try and eat proper portions for a week and see how she feels.

That wasn't hard, right? But let's consider it more carefully. How confident can Patricia feel that in making that simple change, she will discover that she doesn't feel less happy at all, that she doesn't feel confined? Hard to say. Maybe she will. Maybe she won't. Remember, the goal is to give the world a fair chance, even a best shot, to show that the BA we are testing is in some way "off." Patricia's goal is to find out if there is some way that she could feel perfectly happy and not at all confined. So, is there any way to add to or change this test that will make it even more likely that she'll feel that way? Here are some ideas Patricia could incorporate into her test design, as she would write them in the second column of her test design template:

- I will make sure that every meal I eat is made with high-quality, fresh, and healthy ingredients. Does that lead me to feel satisfied eating properly sized portions?

- Every day, I will allow myself half a portion of one "indulgent" food – such as a healthy dessert or snack. Does that lead me to feel satisfied eating properly sized portions?

- I will eat slowly and mindfully, paying attention to how my food looks, feels, and tastes. Does that lead me to feel satisfied eating properly sized portions?

- I will stop after eating a healthy-sized portion and assess how I feel. I will assess how I feel again 20 minutes after the meal. Does that lead me to feel satisfied eating properly sized portions?

After making these additions to her test, Patricia will have increased the chances she will discover she doesn't feel less happy at all and that she doesn't feel confined. Whatever test you design, challenge yourself to increase the chances that you will be able to find that your Big Assumption is not 100% right.

Use S.M.A.R.T. Criteria to Design Your Test

A good test design meets what we call the ***"S-M-A-R-T criteria."*** We'll tell you about the S-M-A parts first and then get to the R-T parts in a bit.

S-M: it is important that your experiment be both **safe** and **modest**. Safe means that if the worst case outcome were to occur, you could live with it. Modest means that the test is relatively easy to carry out. Ideally, it doesn't require you to go out of your way at all, but rather is an opportunity to do something different in your normal day. Safe can also mean you make a *small* change in what you do. Eating smaller portions for a short interval, like a week, is probably safe enough and modest enough for most people to try. Less safe options might be starting a fast, going on a diet that severely restricts you, or confronting your spouse about a long-standing issue that you think somehow stresses you to overeat. Less modest options might be preparing every single meal you eat from scratch, completing a two hour gym session each day, or teaching your kids to cook so that they will take on all of the food preparation responsibilities.

A: a good test will be **actionable** in the near term. You should be able to carry it out within the next week or so. You can easily imagine a setting or upcoming situation in which to run your test. In fact, you may already have begun to make the changes that will test your Big Assumptions.

If your BA focuses on deeper, underlying issues (regarding control, or self-worth, or self-image) you may have to work harder to design a test that is actionable. For example, a test that is designed to be run once you find a new job is probably not very actionable. A test that is designed to be run while you are currently looking for a new job probably is.

Question 2: How are you going to test it? What will you actually do differently (that is safe, modest, and actionable) that will give you good information about the accuracy of your Big Assumption?

Start with the end in mind: what *data* would lead you to doubt your Big Assumption? What type of information (about how you feel or what would happen) would you want to have that would lead you to see that your Big Assumption is not 100% true? Work backwards from there to figure out what safe and modest action you could take in the next week or two that could generate that data. If this suggestion is confusing for you, read ahead to the section titled "Collecting Good Data" and see if that helps you when you come back to this one. If you can't imagine what data could challenge or cast doubt on your assumption, then you don't have a testable assumption. If you are working with a partner, ask for help in rewording your assumptions so that you can test them.
If you still can't come up with a test idea by starting with your Big Assumption, start from a different place. What *behavior* could you change (start or stop doing) that would get you useful information about the accuracy of your Big Assumption?

You could:

- Change one of the behaviors you listed in Column 2 (Doing and Not Doing) of your ITC map

- Do something that runs counter to your Column 3 hidden commitment

- Look at your Picture of Progress and choose to do something that will move you further along

- Look at natural experiments that you experienced during your self-observation exercises and that allowed you to revisit your Big Assumptions. Try an intentional version of one of these.

Sometimes you can come up with a test idea by looking at your calendar to see if there are important events that are ripe for running a test. For example, see if there is an event coming up such as a meeting, family reunion, holiday, interview, or the like that may inspire you to think about ways to behave differently in that event and gather valuable information about your Big Assumption. That will ensure that your test is actionable, but just make sure that what you are planning to do is safe enough, and that you aren't attempting to make too big a change, too quickly. After all, this is just your *first* test.

Now for the **R-T** part of our S-M-A-R-T criteria. A good experiment informally **researches** the question, "how accurate is my Big Assumption?" It also truly ***tests*** the Big Assumption, giving you a reasonable shot at finding out that your Big Assumption is not always right. Like any good research, it requires collecting good data. Your data includes what you say and do differently, as well as what happens as a result. Your feelings can also be a very rich data source. Your test should not be just a clever way to prove that you have been right all along and your Big Assumption is completely true! You may feel some pride in having been right, but you'll end up no closer to overturning your immunity and making progress on your improvement goal.

Collecting Good Data

You should design your test to reveal information that could cast doubt on your assumptions or prove them wrong, if that is the case. For example, remember Patricia? Let's imagine a test to challenge her Big Assumption: "I will feel less happy and more confined if I limit my eating to 'proper portions.'" In running that test, Patricia would need to be very careful to collect *data about whether or not she actually does eat proper portions, and how she feels, of course, when she does*. Did she weigh or otherwise measure her food? Did she cook with healthy and fresh ingredients? Does she allow herself a half-portion of a healthy dessert each day? Does she eat slowly and mindfully? And so on. And, of course, how does she find herself feeling in each situation?

The best quality data will be ***directly observable*** – the actual things people say or do, the words or action that would be captured on a videotape if the event were recorded. This includes what you did and said, as well as what the other people in the test situation did and said. Just as important, however, is experiential data about what you are thinking and feeling as you run your test.

The best way for Patricia to collect her data might be to keep a food diary, listing what and how much she eats every day, along with notes on her eating behaviors and her feelings. Since her Big Assumption is focused on how she would feel, she should record how she actually does feel before, during, and after running all the various parts of this test. She could record all of this information in specially designated sections in her food diary.

Depending on the Big Assumption, you may only be able to collect data about your thinking and feeling. For example, imagine this was your Big Assumption: "I assume that if I feel sympathy for my mother when she offers me second helpings, I will lose touch with my own feelings." Any test designed around this Big Assumption will collect data about your own internal experience (data about your feelings of sympathy and data about whether or not you lose touch with your own feelings). As you collect this type of data, you may notice that you experience many feelings at once, and your feelings may change throughout the test. So try to tune in to your emotions frequently.

"Reading between the lines," or trying to guess what someone else is thinking or feeling is *not good data*. It is easy to slip from noticing another person's reactions to interpreting them. For example, reporting that "my mother did not like what I said when I refused seconds" is not data. "My mother frowned, groaned, and looked away" is good data because it is directly observable: something that was said or done that could be captured if the situation was being videotaped. Try to observe with as little judgment as possible. If data about others' thoughts and feelings are important to the test, you should ask directly for that feedback.

There are usually two parts to a test – what you say or do differently, and the results or outcomes of this new behavior. Try to collect data about both parts. For example, imagine your Big Assumption is "if I ask for help to reduce my stress, people will let me down." Notice what you actually say when you ask for help. If you say, "I'm so busy," hoping that someone will somehow get the hint that you need help, you may get a different result than if you said instead, "Can you help me finish this project?" You'll also need to collect data about the outcomes of your new behavior. What data will indicate whether people let you down or not? Do they offer or agree to help? Do they offer to help but then don't follow through? Do they smile, pat your shoulder, and wish you luck? Getting good data about what you did and what happened will help you learn the most about your Big Assumption.

One way to improve the quality of the data is to enlist others as data collectors. The stronger the grip of your Big Assumption, the less skillful you will be at collecting data and interpreting it accurately. You will have a strong tendency to see things as you want them to be, fear them to be, and/or expect them to be. Getting even one more perspective about the actual data, what it shows, and how it reflects back on the Big Assumption can lead to much more powerful learning.

If you're working with a partner, consider gathering data for each other. If you can include others as data collectors, let them know what you are doing and what kind of data you'd like to collect. Don't choose someone you think might not be honest with you. For example, someone who holds a grudge against you may be biased to see only negative data. A supportive friend or colleague can often be a good choice, as long that person isn't likely to focus only on protecting you and rooting for your success so much that the data is only positive.

Question 3: What data do you plan to collect? Is there anyone to whom you'd like to give a "heads-up" or ask to serve as an observer who can help you collect data or give you feedback after the fact?

Question 4: How will that data help you to confirm or disconfirm your Big Assumption? What results would lead you to think that your BA may not be accurate?

Before you run your test, review your plan using the S-M-A-R-T criteria. It is best to actually evaluate a design, once you have come up with one, "in reverse." (Think "T-R-A-M-S." Start with the "T" and then move to the "R," "A," "M," and then "S.") In other words: What Big Assumption are you testing? What kind of data are you looking for? Can you run this experiment in a week? Will it be effective in testing your BA? Is it simple enough? Finally, is it safe enough?

You should then consider other things you might do to increase your odds of running a successful test. Here are some suggestions:

- **Prepare notes for your test.** Write down what you plan to say and do. Ask your partner to help you practice saying things out loud or behaving differently. Or, if you're working on your own, practice by yourself. Imagine yourself eating differently, exercising regularly, or doing whatever you have planned for your test. Close your eyes and picture each step in the process.

- **Think about how you will respond** to any negative thoughts or voices you hear inside your head. Practice techniques for eliminating negative mind chatter.

- **Imagine different scenarios** for how your test will go and consider how you might want to respond.

    - If you are planning to say something differently, consider the implications of tone of voice, body language, or choice of words. Anticipate how your typical ways of saying things might lead to a foregone conclusion and consider whether there is a more productive approach you could take.

- If you are planning to do something differently, be prepared with alternative strategies for handling responses that might be negative triggers for you.

Sometimes people end up running unplanned tests: life sometimes offers them without warning. Where you are confronted with a situation and suddenly see that you have choices to respond differently than you have in the past, it can be instructive to try something new. These impromptu tests can reveal useful insights about your Big Assumptions.

Nevertheless, we usually find that planned tests offer the most powerful learning for a couple of key reasons. The careful design makes it more likely that you will generate the exact information you are looking for *and* that the information is more likely to be of good quality. That doesn't mean you should never run an unplanned test, but it does mean you should also be devoting most of your attention and work to the ones you plan.

Ron's First Test

Ron thought about all his friends to see if he would feel safe telling any of them about how he was hoping to change. He realized that Don would be a pretty good choice – when Don had to quit smoking to improve his own health, he had been open with Ron about how hard that was. Not only was Don likely to understand why Ron wanted to change his habits, he also would be a good source of support and accountability. Ron realized it would actually be harder to continue to eat poorly if he knew Don was aware of his improvement goal.

Ron's First Test

My Big Assumption Says:	So I will (Change my Behavior This Way)...	And collect the following data ...	In Order to Find Out Whether ...
I assume (no matter what my friends do) that I'll feel less a part of things if I am not eating like my friends are eating.	I'll tell my buddy Don that I'm trying to get healthier by cutting out desserts and snacks. The reason I am telling him is so that it will be harder for me to fall short, so I'll tell him to be watching me. I will cut out all desserts and snacks for two weeks. If someone offers me a dessert or snack, I will say "no thank you."	What does Don say and do? Does he treat me like I'm weird and avoid me or try to talk me out of it? Can I cut out these foods? How will it feel to cut them out? Can I refuse if someone offers me food? How does the person respond? Is there anyone to whom you'd like to give a "heads-up" or ask to serve as an observer who can give you feedback after the fact? No	Don is willing to help me. I can count on him to help me. If I can, and he does help me, do I like that he is helping me? I feel weird saying no to offers.

Miriam's First Test

Miriam told us about the BA she was exploring: "'I assume if I don't criticize myself harshly, I'll slack off too much.' But can see now that criticizing myself actually isn't helping me *at all*. Focusing on how I'm screwing up just makes me feel worse and worse. So can I change that? And if I do stop being so critical of myself, what happens?"

Miriam's First Test

My Big Assumption Says:	So I will (Change my Behavior This Way)…	And collect the following data …	In Order to Find Out Whether …
I assume that if I don't criticize myself harshly, I'll slack off too much.	For the next two weeks, I will spend 15 minutes meditating on my vision for Full Success from my Picture of Progress – trying to feel the details of that picture. I will do this every morning when I wake up. I will keep a copy of my POP in my nightstand next to the bed. I will also keep a copy in my planner. That way I can refer to it if I need help in picturing Full Success. I will cut out all desserts and snacks for two weeks. Throughout the day, I will watch myself very carefully to notice when I start to create and dwell on negative messages about me. When I catch myself going negative, I will remind myself of (or meditate on) where I would like to be – Full Success and try to reconnect with that vision.	How do I feel in the morning when I meditate, when I interrupt myself from a negative interpretation, when I develop a plausible positive one? What kinds of situations are most likely to lead me to start developing negative interpretations? What happens when I identify what type of hunger I am feeling? Is there anyone to whom you'd like to give a "heads-up" or ask to serve as an observer who can give you feedback after the fact? No. Since most of what I am doing happens inside my head, I don't think others will be useful in giving me feedback.	I can develop plausible positive interpretations about myself and what I am doing. Do meditation and reminders help me remember and believe in this possibility? How hard is it to return to and believe in the image of Full Success? Does that image still feel powerful to me? Does it help me feel calm and hopeful?

Clyde's Tests

Clyde had been trying to lose weight for several years, and he was often successful – losing 15 or 20 pounds each time he tried. But each time he lost that weight, he regained it again, sometimes even gaining more than he had taken off. This pattern had repeated itself enough that Clyde was quite aware of the very things that he needed to do to lose weight. He knew how to change his eating. He knew how to work exercise into his daily routine. He even knew how to keep his motivation high by rewarding himself with self-praise and encouragement whenever he lost a few pounds.

He also knew one of the big obstacles in his path had been the ways his wife, Bev, responded to his efforts to lose weight. Bev also wanted to lose weight and announced that she intended to change her habits too. She offered to cook healthier meals and vowed to cut back on her portions. She asked Clyde to let her know when he would go out for a walk in the evenings so that she could join him too. Clyde always tried to be enthusiastic when Bev said she'd join him. He hoped she would start making the same changes he was making. He imagined what it would be like if they could both be successful.

However, whenever Bev declared her intentions to join him, Clyde also felt strong feelings of dread. In the past, Bev had less success changing her diet and exercise habits than he had. She'd start out strong, but then predictably, she would lose her motivation. It just seemed much harder for her to lose weight than it was for Clyde. He'd take off 5 or 10 pounds, and she would get stuck at 2. He found it pretty easy to cut out the evening snacking that they usually did while they watched TV. She couldn't stop thinking about the ice cream in the freezer or the microwave popcorn in the pantry. "Maybe I'll just have a small bowl of yogurt instead," she'd say to Clyde. "Are you sure you don't want some? It's better not to cut back ***too much*** you know, or you'll start to feel deprived. And don't forget that we need to get enough calcium now that we're getting older."

It was hard for Bev to stick to their plan, and it seemed it was even harder for her to watch Clyde succeeding. Invariably, Bev would start to get more and more upset with Clyde as he lost weight, and Clyde would begin to feel that it was harder and harder for them to get along. He would start to feel as though his success was a punishment to Bev, that he was being disloyal and selfish for continuing to succeed. All of these issues made their way into his immunity map, resulting in the following Big Assumption: **"I assume if I lose weight, Bev will go into a deep depression."**

The immunity map and especially his Big Assumptions certainly laid out his problem, and Clyde knew that if he were ever to make meaningful changes in his life, something would have to change in his relationship with Bev. But he was actually feeling pretty pessimistic about the chances that he would discover that Big Assumption was not 100% true. He really didn't want to find out that improving his health would necessarily take a toll on his relationship, and he couldn't figure out how he would ever get a result that would be any different.

So Clyde began to see that his Big Assumption, while powerful, was not actually testable in its current form. He thought carefully about what was most powerful to him about that BA and decided it was the idea of upsetting or disturbing his relationship with his wife. Trying to capture this fear, he wrote, **"I assume my losing weight would be threatening and disturbing to my wife."** That captured the power of his fears but also provided him with a safer way to test – he could start by asking Bev about how she would feel.

That week, Clyde spoke with Bev about his hopes to lose weight and his fears of how she might react. Bev was quiet for a long time but finally told Clyde that she couldn't promise that she would be as supportive and excited as he'd like her to be (and as *she* would actually like to be), but she really wanted them both to try. "I would feel worse, Clyde, if I was the one holding you back. So, I might feel uncomfortable, and I might not be the best support, and I might even try to work on my own weight. But I really want you to do whatever you need to do. And I promise I will be OK."

Clyde was reassured by this conversation, although he still worried that Bev might have a harder time living up to her promises than she thought. Finally, he decided that for his first test, he would start walking during his lunch hour. This test seemed like it had at least some chance of succeeding. Bev might still get upset when she noticed that Clyde was losing weight and getting fitter, but she couldn't make plans to join him, since she would be at work herself at that time. And if she wasn't part of his plan in the first place, that meant that she wouldn't be able to sabotage the plan by backing out and then making Clyde feel he shouldn't carry on either.

Clyde ran this test and felt that he was getting some good results. He was walking regularly and was pleased to start feeling fitter. Bev did make comments about this change in his routine, and some of these comments felt kind of unsupportive to Clyde's goals. "She'll say she doesn't understand why we don't walk together in the evenings since she would like to lose weight too. I feel like her feelings are hurt, like my walking without her makes her feel like I don't want to do it with her or don't want her to get fitter too. And I start to feel twinges of guilt and feel kind of nervous that she'll get even

more upset if I continue." But Clyde was also finding that he did continue. None of the comments Bev was making led to arguments or tears. And while Clyde felt very nervous whenever the subject of his walks came up, he found that he was getting less nervous over time.

That result was very intriguing to Clyde and so he decided he was ready to run a more ambitious test. He also realized after running his test that he had been holding another Big Assumption that was linked to the first one **(I assume that if I pursue proper eating and exercise, Bev will go into a tailspin, or it will create big problems in our relationship.)** Clyde thought about his new assumption and added, **"I also assume that if Bev doesn't support my goals of proper eating and exercise, she will cause a disruption, and *I will not be able to handle her anxiety, disappointment, and jealousy.*"** Thinking back on his earlier attempts to lose weight and exercise, Clyde realized that as soon as Bev had started having trouble herself and making comments to him, he had not followed through on his own plans. He had never tried very hard to maintain his commitments to see what would happen because he simply assumed he would feel too disloyal and experience too much tension between them. This became the focus of his new test design:

Clyde's First Test

My Big Assumption Says:	So I will (Change my Behavior This Way)…	And collect the following data …	In Order to Find Out Whether …
I assume that if I pursue proper eating and exercise, Bev will go into a tailspin, or it will create big problems in our relationship. I also assume that if Bev doesn't support my goals of proper eating and exercise, she will cause a disruption, and I will not be able to handle her own anxiety, disappointment, and jealousy.	I will change my routine back so that I am doing my walking in the evenning after dinner. That way I will also be able to eat a better lunch because I will have more time. I will tell Bev about my change of plans and invite her to come with me on the walks if she wants to. If Bev days she'll come but then doesn't, I will nt stay home with her as I have in the past. Instead, I will take a walk by myself.	How does Bev react? How do I feel about her reaction?	Bev responds as she has in the past - by cancelling and then getting upset. I am able to tolerate Bev's discomfort and anxiety. I am able to make my decision about walking based on my own goals and not her reaction.

As Clyde got ready to run his test he was surprised to realize that he was not feeling very worried about how it would go. "In a way," he explained, "I'm almost hoping that she decides not to go on the walk with me so that I have a chance to see if I can, in fact, not be swayed by what she does." What he realized was that his ability to look to his own goals to make his decision meant far more to him than simply whether or not he ended up going for a walk. And so, by the time he actually ran his test, Clyde was not surprised by the results.

"It was completely fine," he reflected. "Bev opted out of our walk at the last minute, and I told her I thought I'd go anyway. She was really surprised. I think I kind of shocked her. But I felt pretty calm inside, and I just smiled at her and said that I'd be back soon, and I went. Everything has been different since then. I think Bev is kind of adjusting to the idea that I am going to go for my walk, with her or without her. And I bet she is feeling some anxiety herself about this whole thing. But it hasn't been awful at all – she makes some comments and thinks of reasons sometimes why walking isn't a good idea, and that's OK. It's still my decision, and so I go by myself. And what I notice is that I'm happier. I'm not as focused on what she'll do and how she'll react, and that means I'm less worried because what I do is not dependent on what she does or how she feels. And that feels really good. And so when I come home from my walk, I'm in a great mood. And then we can relax together and talk about our days and watch TV.

"I think there might be some truth to my first assumption. Bev might have a negative reaction still to my progress, although it hasn't been anything like a tailspin. But my second assumption is not true. I have learned that I can handle her disappointment and anxiety. I can deal with her making comments that might have undermined me before. I might still feel some twinges of disloyalty at times and worry that my choices are having a negative impact on her and on our relationship. But more than all that, I've seen that I can do things that are really important to me, and the benefits to that far outweigh the negatives. I feel great. I feel great about me, and I feel great about my marriage with Bev. And I never would have believed that these changes were really possible until now."

9

Running And Interpreting Your Tests

I've disconnected food from my feelings. I know I don't have to eat to be social. I am no longer turning to food when I feel stressed and am finding a new way to deal with the stress. Immunity to Change has been a really good thing for me. I didn't think I'd say that. I started off encouraged, but as it got harder, then I thought I'd need to quit because I was worried I wouldn't do it perfectly. But that was actually my Big Assumption, "If I can't do something perfectly, I should stop. I shouldn't do it." I was starting to play that assumption out, but then it just jumped out at me, and I understood what I was doing! Wanting to quit ITC was just another example of the BA "I'm not going to do it at all if I can't do it perfectly."

Deep down I've known a lot of this stuff mentally, but I haven't been willing to let go of those fears and BAs. By being able to focus through these small tests, I had that opportunity to really question them. It's one thing to feel you know something isn't true and another to actually believe it about yourself.

— Dana

Finally, your test is ready! Go ahead and run it, and make sure you have a good way to keep track of what happens, such as by taking written notes. Basically, you'll want to record what you actually did, what happened as a result, and what you felt and thought about it. You'll find this exercise in the "Running and Interpreting Tests" portion of your Change Journal.

1. Write your Big Assumption.

2. Then write what you actually did to test your Big Assumption. This may be what you planned to do (in which case you can simply copy the text from your test design) or you may have done something else (which is fine!).

3. Write what you observed happening. This includes what you saw and heard other people do or say, as well as what you were feeling.

4. Write what you learned about the accuracy of your Big Assumption.

Interpreting Your Test Data

So, did you run a good test? Were you able to behave differently than you usually do? Sometimes you don't end up running the exact test you planned, but you still learn important information about your Big Assumption. If you feel like your test was too flawed to be useful, no problem. You may still be able to run the test you had originally planned, or you can design a new one. If you conclude that the test you ran was sound, you are ready to look at your data for the sole purpose of understanding what it suggests about your Big Assumption. **Remember, the purpose of running a good test is not to see whether you improved, i.e., whether your behavior change "worked" (although this is not unimportant), but rather to use the test results to inform your Big Assumption.** As we keep saying, a big difference in this approach is that we are taking action *not* to get better (immediately), but to get *information*. You will know you are on track if you can see what aspects of your Big Assumption, if any, are confirmed by the data, and what aspects, if any, are disconfirmed, or at least questionable.

When you begin to interpret your data, you may be more likely to see the information that confirms your Big Assumption, and not the information that casts doubt on it. You may quickly focus on the ways your data supports your Big Assumption and not consider other ways you could be interpreting that very same data. Big Assumptions that have a powerful hold tend to direct our attention to whatever will keep them alive and well. So, we suggest that you try to imagine at least one other way that you could be interpreting your data. (If nothing comes to mind, try this: imagine someone else, a real person, who happened to be in that exact situation, and the same things happened. How might you show this person how the results cast some doubt on his or her Big Assumption? If that doesn't get you anywhere, and you are working with a partner, ask him or her to offer an interpretation. Otherwise, find a person you trust to suggest his or her interpretation.)

Creating other interpretations is especially important if you feel your test did not go as well as you had hoped. Maybe you weren't able to change your behavior; others didn't welcome the new behaviors; or your new behaviors didn't lead to the hoped-for results. You may even be disappointed to learn that your Big Assumption seems to be accurate in the particular context in which you ran your test. But all of these scenarios can still help you learn about your Big Assumption – under what conditions it is and isn't accurate. And they can also suggest ideas for new tests.

Here is an example of how generating alternative interpretations can be useful to overall progress. Jason's Big Assumption was that following healthy eating habits would be boring and would make his life feel too routine. He was used to "life in the fast lane," where he and his wife were always out at parties, meeting friends for drinks, or trying out a new local restaurant together. To test his assumption that being healthier meant giving up fun and excitement, he planned to start a support group for people he knew who were also trying to eat healthier and exercise. He imagined they could plan lots of fun activities together – like long biking and hiking trips. He looked into hiring a fitness instructor to come and give the group individualized workout sessions. He contacted a friend who loved cooking and asked her if she would cater a "healthy summer fun" party that would feature smoothies, low-calorie snacks, and include recipes that they could all try to make themselves at home. As Jason developed these plans, he got very excited about the possibilities that a healthier lifestyle could still be as full and exciting as he wanted.

But two weeks later, he was annoyed and disappointed when two couples emailed him to say that they couldn't come to the party, and that they would not be able to participate in all of the group activities Jason was planning. Jason worried that his test was now failing and that his plans for a healthy, but still exciting new lifestyle might not be possible. What should he do? Give up? Work even harder? Design a new test? As he was explaining his predicament to his wife, he admitted, "I was starting to think that my Big Assumption was true and that it was just going to be too hard to keep this up. I'd either end up living a dull but healthy life, or I'd go back to all my old habits, just so I could have some fun again!"

Jason's wife suggested that he get back in touch with the two couples who had cancelled to see why their initial enthusiasm for the group had changed. Jason agreed, and what he found out gave him a completely different interpretation of his test results. Both couples explained that they were still very enthusiastic about the idea of a healthy lifestyle support group, but they were concerned that Jason's plans were going to end up costing a lot more money than they were willing to spend on parties and trips. To them, it sounded like Jason was going to expect everyone to be paying quite a bit to participate in all the activities he was planning.

"Well, I wasn't thrilled to hear that," Jason later explained. "I mean, it is much easier to have fun if you're willing to spend a little money. But, I do see their point." He paused for a moment and then added, "I mean, really though, I was whipping up all these elaborate plans because I was so excited by the possibility that living more healthily could still be fun, but I didn't need all those things to happen *right away*. So, we worked out a more reasonable budget, and as a group, we try to do something once a month or so. And not everyone has to do everything."

Jason continued, "In terms of that test, my wife helped me see that I was making an interpretation that the test was failing and my Big Assumption was true without really exploring whether that was actually the case. It wasn't the case. I just kind of panicked at the thought that my plans might not work out perfectly and then thought NOTHING would work." As Jason learned, it can be hard to think clearly and calmly during a test of a Big Assumption. Remembering to look for other ways of interpreting your data can lead you to develop more reliable conclusions.

Sometimes, even when a test goes well and allows the person to redefine her Big Assumptions, it is not because she necessarily got only positive results. For example, Amy was running tests on the following Big Assumption: "I assume that eating less, eating only healthy foods, and having to plan my meals will feel *boring* and will be *too much hard work*." Over the course of about six weeks, Amy ran several tests in which she made and brought her home-cooked, healthy lunch to work every day and was cooking healthier meals at home for her family. She had been reading several food blogs that offered nutritional guidance and healthy recipes, and she was surprised to find out how much she was learning and how interesting the subject of nutrition and food preparation had become to her. She was even more excited that she was losing weight, and none of her old clothes were fitting anymore. Now she had an excuse to go shopping after work and was so proud to be wearing smaller sizes. Her Big Assumption – that she would be bored and feel she was working too hard – seemed silly to her now. On the contrary, she could hardly contain her excitement and pride.

Amy's test was designed to gather information about whether she would feel bored or that she was working too hard. Her test enabled her to collect data that cast doubt on her Big Assumption. Unfortunately, her test also produced a different result in that Amy's family and co-workers were less than supportive. Rather than sharing her excitement about her new cooking and eating habits, her new learning about nutrition, and her new, smaller-sized wardrobe, they seemed mostly annoyed. Her children complained that they missed the meals they were used to having. They rolled their eyes when Amy started explaining about the nutritional content of their meals. Her co-workers stopped complimenting her on her weight loss and new clothes and began cutting her off when she brought up the subject of her weight loss success. Amy was puzzled. Why wasn't her family more interested in eating healthy? Couldn't they see how much difference it had made for her? Were her co-workers jealous of her success? Why weren't people more excited for her? Amy felt hurt. Did people really want her to go back to the way she was before? "My test was a disaster!" she told us.

You may already be developing your own interpretations about what was happening in these situations. Maybe Amy's excitement sounded too much like bragging to her coworkers. Maybe her children actually *were* proud of her but *weren't* excited to have to change their eating habits too. Maybe her coworkers actually were jealous of her success and so were finding it hard to be as supportive as she wanted them to be.

But whatever is going on, the first thing Amy needed to be clear about was this: from an ITC perspective, her test was anything but a disaster! It helped her take a big step away from a constraining Big Assumption, which is huge progress! The idea that she would feel bored or work too hard in changing her diet had almost no power anymore. It's true she was also experiencing some unexpected fallout in the wake of her success, and she would need to look into this and decide what to do about it, but this fallout is actually a whole different issue that has no bearing on the ITC results of her particular experiments.

Ron Interprets His First Test Data

My Big Assumption says:

I assume (no matter what my friends do) that I'll feel less a part of things if I am not eating like my friends are eating. I will feel like I am missing out on the full experience.

So in order to test it I changed my behavior this way:

I told Don that I'm trying to get healthier by cutting out desserts and snacks. I told him to be watching me so I don't screw up.

I cut out desserts and snacks for two weeks.

This is what I observed happening:

Telling Don was pretty easy. He agreed to help and then asked me what he should do if he caught me screwing up. He started making lots of jokes about stuff he could do or say – pretty ridiculous ideas – and that got me a little nervous. I was afraid that I had just asked him to make me look like an idiot, basically. I let him joke for a while, but then I got more serious and said how about if I had to give him $5 for each time he caught me. But he couldn't tell anyone or all bets are off. So he said OK. I probably should have thought about all this before I talked to him, but then I think it worked out OK. And there is no way I was going to give him $5, so I didn't screw up even once.
Nobody offered me food, but I really made sure that didn't happen. I ate at my desk instead of eating at the cafeteria at work. There weren't any parties or anything like that at work. I guess the only place I had to turn down a snack was at home. Obviously, my wife and kids know I'm cutting back. They were easy to tell and really want me to get healthier. So nobody suggested we go out to eat, and my wife gave kids dessert after I left the table. Just one day my kids offered me some of their Pop Tarts because they know I like them. But I had already eaten breakfast, so it would have been a snack. I just said, "That's a snack! Can't do it!" And we all laughed.

This is what the data tells me about my Big Assumption:

It was fine to tell Don, and I don't think he is treating me weird. I mean, I guess with him at least, I can feel like things are the same. I didn't feel "not a part." Even goofing with me about what he would do – that's a lot better than if he kind of took it too seriously or tried to talk me out of it or something. I knew Don would be the easiest friend to tell, and how that all went makes me think I could probably tell the others.

And, I learned I can avoid the offers of food if I want. I didn't feel I was missing out on anything. When I started to write down what I learned from this test, I was kind of proud of avoiding that. But, the fact that I didn't have to refuse any offers, unless you count my daughters, is only because I avoided the whole thing. I don't know how long I can keep that up because somebody is going to offer me food, and also, I don't really like eating at my desk every day, which makes me feel strange. So, I have to try harder on being in situations where I get offered food and learn to say no.

Miriam Interprets Her Test Data

My Big Assumption says:

I assume that if I don't criticize myself harshly, I'll slack off too much.

So in order to test it I changed my behavior this way:

Every morning I meditated on my vision for Full Success from my POP – trying to feel the details of that picture.

I made sure I always had a copy of my POP nearby, and I did refer to it sometimes – especially when my head was starting to spin.
I really made the effort to watch myself and notice when I was creating and dwelling on negative messages about me. Sometimes I could catch myself right away, but there were a couple of times when I didn't catch myself until much later.

When I did catch myself going negative, I reminded myself of (or meditated on) where I would like to be — Full Success — and tried to reconnect with that vision. Usually I could create at least one alternative interpretation that was more positive and still felt valid.

Instead of criticizing myself, when I felt hungry, I tried to pause to identify my true feelings – hunger for food or emotional hunger or discomfort?

This is what I observed happening:

I was running late to a meeting, and then when I did get there, I was still kind of mad at myself for being late. I realized, though, that by focusing on what I had done wrong, I wasn't paying attention to what was being said at the meeting. In a way, I was making myself even later. That could make me even madder, but I stopped myself in my head and said, "It's over. You're here now. Be here now. Breathe." It's not really a "positive" interpretation, but repeating that to myself was sort of soothing and calmed me down enough to listen. And then later, after the meeting, I felt good that I had been able to calm down and concentrate. This kind of thing is exciting to me!

The POP helped me think of positive things. The lines "I feel good about myself, I value my own opinions, I feel at ease in my own skin, I feel whole" really help. They are like a mantra. When I say them to myself, I say them in a slow rhythm, and I imagine that I'm sitting cross-legged, breathing deeply, with my eyes closed like I do when I'm meditating. That calms me down and I start to feel better.

When I felt hungry (which was ALWAYS), I tried to pause to identify my true feelings – hunger for food or emotional hunger or discomfort? I wasn't very good at this – it was really hard because the feelings were so uncomfortable, and I had this inner voice screaming at me, "EAT SOMETHING NOW!"

The busier and more stressed I was, the harder it was to make myself pause and take a breath. I felt like, "I don't have time to interrupt myself!" I need to keep working on this.

Where I failed: I had a fight with Paul (my husband) because he feels like I'm letting too many things slide at home. I forgot that my daughter needed a new backpack, so she has been just carrying stuff in her arms. She's pretty mad about that. Also, I am behind on the laundry, and the bathrooms need cleaning, etc. AND we had to go out twice last week in the evening for Paul's job. He thought I seemed tired and not enthusiastic enough to go to these and says I should be more supportive. It was a ton of stuff to dump on me, and we yelled about it for a while. I felt terrible – guilty and lazy and mad at myself for not paying more attention to these things. I was mad at him too, and then later felt like I shouldn't have gotten so mad... and only as I was lying in bed fuming later that night did I think about how I was being negative. And it was too hard to stop myself and try to come up with other interpretations. I was too tired but also too upset to sleep. I got up and went to the kitchen and made myself some hot milk and cookies. This started me on even more negative thinking about myself. Then finally, after I had eaten about four cookies, I froze and said (out loud), "STOP IT NOW!" It was so weird to be yelling at myself like that.
I was telling myself to stop eating, but I was also telling myself to stop working myself up even more. That's what I was doing – just making everything worse. I forced myself to get up and go into another room. For some reason, I picked the bathroom. And I just sat down on the floor next to the bathtub and made myself take several deep breaths. Finally, I felt ready to meditate. I pictured my POP, but thoughts about our fight kept breaking in. After 20 minutes, I was so tired, I went to bed.

So, that was kind of a terrible thing, although if I weren't running this test, it probably would have been much worse. I would have just kept eating and eating and making myself feel even more terrible with self-punishment and blame.

Overall, I would say I feel much more... even. The highs and lows and stress and tiredness feel like they are evening out more. I am calmer and more focused, although it is hard work to be watching myself and working to stay in the right mental space all the time. I know I need to keep doing this, but I hope it gets easier.

This is what the data tells me about my big assumption:

My assumption feels mostly wrong now. When I start criticizing myself, I just feel worse and then there is like a spiral downward. I lose control and binge, or I can't focus because my head is spinning with self-punishment, and I can't stand that feeling anymore.

But even though I know it is wrong, this is going to be hard to change how I see myself. I've been thinking that way for most of my life. And especially when things aren't going well and I'm fighting with Paul or when I do screw up at work, it is just so easy to see only the negative.

I need to keep working on developing more plausible positive interpretations about myself and what I'm doing. Sometimes I don't even think it has to be positive. I just have to calm down and feel balanced again and let go of the negative. The good news is I was able to do this much more than I thought I could. So that helps a lot. Meditation definitely helps, although after that fight, I had to calm down a lot before I could even meditate.

The image of Full Success does still feel powerful for me, and the more I return to it, the quicker I can get to that same place that feels more calm and hopeful. Repeating my mantra helps. Calling up the image of myself meditating helps. Even though I've never meditated outside, when I picture myself meditating – I imagine I'm sitting under a tree overlooking a beautiful view of a valley, and the sun is setting, and the air is very calm and still. And then I just relax more, and it feels like someone is very gently placing their hands on my shoulders until the tension in my muscles starts to release. I'm learning that when I can calm down, I'm far more productive than when I criticize myself!

What Else Have You Learned?

After running and interpreting your first test, revisit your Picture of Progress. Have you discovered any new thoughts, feelings or behaviors that you want to add to it? You might also want to look at the next chapter ("Taking Stock"), not because you are finished testing but because many of the questions in that chapter will help you learn even more from the tests you are running. By now, we hope you are starting to learn some very interesting things about your Big Assumption. Remember, Big Assumptions are beliefs that we have been treating as if they are always 100% right, but they are rarely completely and always right or wrong. So, we run tests to find out when we have been relying too much on them and using them when they are not right. Even small changes to a Big Assumption can help overturn your immunities to change.

Running Additional Tests

It is very rare to learn everything you need to know about your Big Assumption from one test. Often, what you learn from your first test will leave you with questions that you can look to answer in your next test, which may even be just a different version of your first one. You may decide to run the same test with a different person or in a different circumstance. You may decide you are ready to run a test that is more ambitious or one that felt too risky to run earlier. The more you run tests, the more you will learn. Even if you only learn a little from each test, the learning will begin to build until you find you have overturned your immunity to change. Once your Big Assumption no longer feels very powerful or very true, you will also see that your self-protective Column 3 commitments are no longer necessary. You will stop needing to generate the obstructive Column 2 behaviors. And you will be making clear and measurable progress on your improvement goal.

What are your thoughts about a *next* test of your Big Assumption? Think about what you have already learned about your Big Assumption. What do you still need to learn about to discover how your Big Assumption might not be 100% true? In your Change Journal, you'll see plenty of space for designing and running additional tests.

Ron Runs More Tests

Ron's next test was simply a more ambitious version of his first test. He decided to let more of his friends and co-workers know that he was trying to eat less and eat healthier. He put himself in situations where someone was likely to have brought food and where he would have to politely decline to eat it to see if he necessarily would feel less a part of things. He kept running this same test over and over for the course of several weeks as various situations presented themselves.

Ron's Second Test

My Big Assumption Says:	So I will (Change my Behavior This Way)...	And collect the following data ...	In Order to Find Out Whether ...
I assume (no matter what my friends do) that I'll feel less a part of things if I am not eating like my friends are eating. I'll feel like I am "missing out" on the full experience.	I will tell more of my friends and co-workers that I am cutting back and eating healthier. I will tell them about the success I have already had (lost 7 pounds so far) and tell them I don't want to get derailed. If I'm at a meeting or party or at the bar, I will really limit my eating/drinking and refuse additional food/drink that people try to give me. Whenever there is group eating like at a meeting or party, I will make up my mind what I'm going to have and how much, and then once that is done, I'll stop. I will also focus on why I am there - to enjoy hanging out with them.	How do people respond when I tell them or when I refuse their food? Can I continue to stick to my plans (no dessert, no snacks), and only eat as much as I have planned to? How will I feel? Do I feel I am not a part, or missing out? **Is there anyone to whom you'd like to give a "heads-up" or ask to serve as an observer who can give you feedback after the fact?** Yeah, since Don already knows, he has kind of been paying attention to how I'm doing. We can talk about this.	People respond to me in good ways. Can I still enjoy being with these people in these type of gatherings if I'm not eating the same way I used to? Do I feel like I'm a part of things?

Ron – Interpretation of test data

My Big Assumption says:

I assume (no matter what my friends do) that I'll feel less a part of things if I am not eating like my friends are eating. And I'll feel I'm missing out on the full experience.

So in order to test it I changed my behavior this way:

I told most of my friends and co-workers that I am cutting back and eating healthier.

I told them about the success I have already had and said I don't want to get derailed.

I am pretty much limiting my eating/drinking at parties and meetings where there is food. But I am focusing on enjoying being with people.

I can sometimes say no when people offer me food.

I do make up my mind what I'm going to have and how much, and then once that is done, I'll usually stop. But sometimes I do eat more. Once, I ate a lot more.

This is what I observed happening:

People have been much more supportive than I thought. For the most part, they congratulate me on my weight loss and offer their support. We had an office meeting last week, and somebody brought in donuts. I really wanted one and felt kind of on-the-spot. When I didn't take one, somebody said, "Oh, you are being so good!" I felt good for refusing instead of bad.

It is hardest with my bar friends. We still go together but I try to drink less and to drink slowly. I don't order a bacon cheeseburger like I did before. I feel pretty aware all the time that I can't just drink like I used to, without thinking about how much I've already had. I do feel uncomfortable, but then I usually feel better later, better than I used to when I would be hung-over and too full. And I notice I pay more attention to our conversations now than I did before!

The time I gave in was last Friday. I was just kind of fed up of working so hard and being so careful, and I drank a couple of beers pretty quickly. Then it was so easy to just drink more and eat and eat. At the time, it felt good – like I could completely let go. But then later I felt terrible of course. And my friends kept ribbing me about "falling off the wagon."

This is what the data tells me about my Big Assumption:

At work I have no problem. The support I am getting from people feels really good, so I don't feel at all strange or like I don't fit in if I am eating well. People actually give me compliments and stuff.

But I think my assumption is actually mostly true when I go to the bar with my friends. I just don't feel comfortable and relaxed like I used to because I am so aware of not drinking or eating too much, and now I can't really enjoy it even if I do. It just isn't the same as it used to be. I'm not sure I feel less a part of things, but I do feel I'm not having the full experience.

Ron's Third Test

My Big Assumption Says:	So I will (Change my Behavior This Way)...	And collect the following data ...	In Order to Find Out Whether ...
I assume (no matter what my friends do) that I'll feel less a part of things if I am not eating like my friends are eating, and I'll feel I'm missing out on the full experience.	I will organize my bar buddies to start playing some ball together after work before we go to the bar. I will try to enjoy and feel part of the game - should be easy.	Do they agree to play? How do I feel? What do they say and do when we're playing? **Is there anyone to whom you'd like to give a "heads-up" or ask to serve as an observer who can give you feedback after the fact?** Actually, Don came up with the idea for this test, so I'm sure he'll be watching to see what happens.	We can have as much fun playing ball together as we do at the bar. I drink less when we go to the bar. I enjoy hanging out with them more than I have been. I continue to lose weight because now I will be getting more exercise.

Ron – Interpretation of Test Data

My Big Assumption says:

I assume (no matter what my friends do) that I'll feel less a part of things if I am not eating like my friends are eating, and I'll feel like I'm missing out on the full experience.

So in order to test it I changed my behavior this way:

I organized a weekly hoops game on Fridays after work. The guys said they'd try it out. I tried to enjoy myself and feel part of the game, which was easy to do.

This is what I observed happening:

The first time, we played for an hour or so on a local court and then went to the bar. The first game we sweated like pigs. But it was fun too, and then we showed up at the bar all sweaty, so nobody actually wanted to stay very long. I felt bad about that. But then we decided to play at the local Y, where we can all shower after. Of course by the time we get to the bar, we're all starving, so we probably still kind of eat more than we should. I do, anyway. But I drink less because I'm just not there for as long as I used to be.

OK, so I think playing hoops can become our new routine, and this thing really may work! I am having a blast, really enjoying hanging out with my friends, and even though I suck at hoops now, I feel better than I did before I started this whole process. And I like it. It's good exercise, and I like hanging out with my friends this way, like we all did when we were in our 20s and still single. I forgot that we used to do that.

This is what the data tells me about my Big Assumption:

I can find better ways of hanging out with my friends and not feeling like I have to be eating and drinking with them. I can still do some of that, and I enjoy it. But now I can see that there are other ways of hanging out together that don't mean we all turn out to be fat drunks. I certainly don't feel I'm less a part of things. As for "missing out on the full experience" I feel two things: (1) when we are hanging out in this new way (hoops) I certainly don't feel I'm missing out on the full experience; (2) when it comes to eating and drinking, I actually don't mind having a little less than the "full experience" because it is a small price to pay for a big reward. I think that what it means to me to have a "full experience" might even be changing too.

Miriam Runs More Tests

Miriam thought about how to keep challenging her Big Assumption. "When I criticize myself and jump into a negative view of myself, I feel terrible. And I hate feeling terrible, so I try to blot out that emotion by eating. Of course that only makes me feel more terrible. So now that I'm seeing that telling myself I'm messed up actually doesn't help, I've been working on not going negative in the first place. I'm still working on this. And it has made me much more aware of my general confusion around my emotions. I think I've been trying to act on or avoid or engineer my emotions for so long that it is hard for me to even know what I'm really feeling. There are many times when even I'm not sure I know what I feel, and if it is a painful feeling, then I just try to run away from it. What is very related to that is being able to stay with my feelings – to be able to name them and withstand them (even when they are negative)."

Miriam's Second Test

My Big Assumption Says:	So I will (Change my Behavior This Way)...	And collect the following data ...	In Order to Find Out Whether ...
I assume that if I don't criticize myself harshly, I'll slack off too much. I realize I have also been assuming that every time I feel stressed or emotional, I must eat to make myself feel better.	I will ask myself to check in and see what I am feeling – to see if I can identify my emotions and allow myself to feel them rather than mislabeling them as "hunger for food" and/or trying to run away from them. If I am feeling something negative (loneliness, stress, fear, etc.), I will consciously remind myself to notice and acknowledge the feeling and tell myself that I will let it pass through me as it needs to. I am bigger than any bad feeling. I can withstand it. I will do these check-ins several times a day, especially when I am about to eat something. I will also keep working to listen to my body to see if I can identify when I am really hungry for food, what food tastes good, and how much my body wants.	What am I feeling? What do I do in response to my emotions? What ways (other than eating) can I use to respond to my emotions? **Is there anyone to whom you'd like to give a "heads-up" or ask to serve as an observer who can give you feedback after the fact?** No – this is really about my own feelings.	I can identify my emotions. I can allow myself to feel a negative emotion without panic or overeating. I can distinguish emotional hunger from physical hunger.

Miriam – Interpretation of Test Data

My Big Assumption says:

I assume that if I don't criticize myself harshly, I'll slack off too much.

I assume that every time I feel stressed or emotional, I must eat to make myself feel better.

So in order to test it I changed my behavior this way:

Every day, I regularly checked (especially when I felt "hungry") to see what I was feeling – to see if I could identify my emotions and allow myself to feel them rather than mislabeling them as "hunger for food" and/or trying to run away from them.

When I was feeling something negative (loneliness, stress, fear, etc.), I consciously reminded myself to notice and acknowledge the feeling and tell myself to let it pass through me as it needs to. ("I am bigger than any bad feeling. I can withstand it.")

I worked to listen to my body to see if I could identify when I was really hungry for food, what food tasted good, and how much my body wanted. When I ate, I tried only to focus on eating.

This is what I observed happening:

Regardless of whether my stomach is actually hungry, I have an urge to eat when I am bored, when I'm working on something that is hard and I feel like I need a break, when the clock says it is time to eat, when I see food, when I see someone else eating, when I've just finished doing something but haven't yet started the next thing, when I'm tired, when I'm too wound up, when I first come home at the end of the day, any time I go into the kitchen, when I finish a meal (I'm already thinking about the next one), when I know that there is tempting food somewhere near me (in the fridge or pantry, next to the coffee pot at work), when I see ads for food, when I smell food, when I am winding down at night.

I became really aware of how wanting to eat something is almost constantly on my mind, whether I'm really hungry or not.

So then I also noticed when it is not on my mind: when I'm busy or really thinking hard about something else, when I'm exercising, when I'm feeling my most calm and happy, when I feel successful. I am starting to see that there is a positive relationship here – just like criticizing and punishing myself leads me to want to eat more, feeling good about myself and in control lead me to feel full and satisfied.

And, it is still kind of rare for me to be in that positive space. So when I was feeling stressed or guilty or frustrated, I just kept telling myself, "That's fine. You won't die from these feelings. Just let them move through you. Breathe deeply." It did help me feel calmer and stronger – I kind of imagined the feeling was coming through me as if it was being pushed through by a light breeze.

Sometimes when I still wanted to eat, I would go brush my teeth, which helped me feel clean and light, like I had just woken up.

This is what the data tells me about my Big Assumption:

I am not my emotions! I can feel them without them taking over and making me feel like I have to eat. They feel less powerful and less scary.

I still have lots of cravings for food that I don't think are really hunger, but I don't just obey them now. I try to reason with them a little to see what I should do about them. I am getting better at distinguishing emotional hunger from physical hunger.

In paying attention to what makes me positive and happy, I keep realizing how much this happens at work. I really do like my work and am starting to feel like I haven't really been giving myself enough credit there. I haven't let myself enjoy it because it made me feel guilty, like I shouldn't like it so much, shouldn't enjoy my successes and shouldn't think about moving up in the organization. This is a big "Aha" for me, and it is a little scary, but I think I'm getting more ambitious!

Miriam was really struck by what she was learning about her feelings toward her work. As she reflected on how much she enjoyed her work, she realized that she had been holding herself back there in large part because she was worried about how her family would react to her ambition. She looked back at her Biography of her Big Assumption and thought about how important it was to her family that she follow the family "script" and not let work interfere with their expectations for her as a wife and mother. She also knew that she had probably been more tentative in setting her own expectations because she feared finding out that she wasn't smart enough. But the feedback she had been getting at work had all been so positive and so encouraging. "I'm getting all these green lights at work, but I'm still moving slowly and cautiously," she saw. "I think I'm still holding myself back because I'm kind of afraid of what I could be. I'm afraid if I don't keep myself small, there will be conflict and chaos in my family." She realized that she had a new Big Assumption to add to her map and to test: "I assume that I must keep myself small and limit my potential in order to preserve love and approval in my family."

"Wow, that means I have *needed* to find faults in myself, to believe something is wrong with me. That has kept me 'safe' if pursuing my dreams would mean that my family and Paul don't really want me to challenge their expectations for me. That's why I was worried about people seeing who I really am and potentially rejecting me. I thought it was because the real me was screwed up, but now I'm thinking that at least part of it was that I was too scared to believe in myself. I was too scared to let others see what I really want because… I don't think they'll like it. I don't think they'll like *me*."

Miriam knew she was ready to test this assumption and felt the safest test would be with her family – with her father in particular. She felt sure of his love, although she was worried that he wouldn't really be able to understand what she was ready to tell him.

Miriam's Third Test

My Big Assumption Says:	So I will (Change my Behavior This Way)…	And collect the following data …	In Order to Find Out Whether …
I assume that if I don't criticize myself harshly, I'll slack off too much. I assume that I must keep myself small and limit my potential in order to preserve love and approval in my family. I assume if people saw the real me, they would reject me.	I will talk to my father and tell him what I think I need to do in order to be truly happy. I will try to understand his perspective – why he has been so strict with me about how he thinks I should be living my life. I will ask him if he thinks he can support me in those goals. I will plan out exactly what I want to say and imagine some different ways he might respond. I will decide how I would like to respond to him in each of these cases.	What do I say to my father? What does he say to me? How do I feel (while I'm planning, during the conversation, afterward)? Is there anyone to whom you'd like to give a "heads-up" or ask to serve as an observer who can give you feedback after the fact? There is a friend of mine from my women's book group. I have been talking to her a little bit about what I am starting to see about my life. I have asked her if I can talk through my plans with her before the conversation and if she will help me debrief the conversation afterward	I can make a case that I truly believe about what I want and communicate this to him. I can bear the possibility of his disapproval without caving in on my own truth. I can minimize the chances of ruining my relationship with him.

Miriam – Interpretation of Test Data

My Big Assumption says:

I assume that if I don't criticize myself harshly, I'll slack off too much.
I assume that I must keep myself small and limit my potential in order to preserve love and approval in my family.
I assume if people saw the real me, they would reject me.

So in order to test it I changed my behavior this way:

I planned out everything I wanted to say in advance and then met with Solange (my book group friend). She reminded me of a book (called Difficult Conversations) that we had read in our book group, and I used that to help me prepare – to focus not just on what I have decided but also on my feelings about all of this, my feelings about my father, and what is at stake for me in this whole issue. I told her everything I planned to say, and then we speculated about the various ways he might react (and how I wanted to respond to him).

Then I made arrangements to have dinner with my father and to tell him that I think I will only be truly happy when I feel like I am fulfilling my potential more at work. I told him that will mean I spend less time at home with the kids. I definitely did most of the talking because I had planned out everything I wanted to tell him... and it was quite a bit. Finally I asked what he was thinking and if he can support me in my goals.

This is what I observed happening:

That planning helped a lot. I felt really nervous for the conversation because I still didn't know how he would react, but I also knew I had done everything I could to help it go well. I knew I had a plan even if my worst fears came true.

After I finally stopped talking, my father was really quiet for a while. He is not a loud or talkative man anyway, but I felt like the pause he took was so long. Then he told me how sad he felt that I had believed he was holding me back. "I never wanted that for you. I just wanted to be happy. And we do the best we can to help our children get all the things that were so hard for us. Having a secure life is something many people don't have, and we didn't always have that in our family. Having a happy family is also fairly rare nowadays, and that is why we tried so hard to help you kids see that as the center of your lives. I was so pleased when you married and started having kids because I knew how happy that made me." Then he didn't say anything for a while. Then he said, "What does Paul think of this?"

My voice started to shake a bit when I told him I was really worried about how Paul will react. My dad didn't say anything. He just kept looking down at the table. Finally, he looked at me again and said, "Well, that's something you'll have to work out with him then. I hope you're not going to throw the whole thing away."

We started talking about my marriage a little, but then I remembered the planning I had done with Solange, where I decided that I didn't want to focus on Paul when I was talking to my dad. I wanted to focus on my relationship with him (my father). So then I said, "Dad, I don't know what will happen with Paul. I promise you I will try my best to make it work. But I don't really want to talk about that with you tonight. What I really want to know from you is if you can support me to pursue my potential." Again, there was a long pause and he said, "Miriam, you are my daughter, and I will always love you. That's about as much as I can say right now."

I felt scared and thrilled pretty much through the whole conversation. I was most scared when I faced how very worried I am about how Paul will react. I've never said that to anyone. In that moment, I realized the possibility that we could be divorced. That was frightening and relieving all at once. I was also very scared when I asked again for my dad's support. But as I was leaving the restaurant, I felt like I had taken a big step forward about believing in myself. That felt so, so, so good. The whole time I was driving home I kept replaying the conversation in my head and taking deep breaths to try and calm myself down.

This is what the data tells me about my Big Assumption:

I learned that I can make a case for what I truly believe about what I want and communicate this to him. I learned that I really want his approval, but I'm also willing to have him disappointed in me if it means I'm staying true to what I think I want. Staying clear about my own goals helped a lot – it showed me how important it really is to me to find out just what my potential is at work. And I feel good about how my dad reacted. I mean, it wasn't perfect, but I think it was really hard for him to say he would support me and just his telling me he loved me was enough. I learned he doesn't want me to keep myself small or limit my potential even if he does worry about where that will lead.

I realize that I need to cross off three of my BAs:

- I assume if I don't criticize myself really harshly, I'll slack off too much.
- I assume that if I try to lose weight, I will actually feel worse, be under more pressure, and I will fail.
- I assume I have even bigger faults than my weight that will keep me unhappy, and if I get thin I will have to face these, and I won't be able to deal with them.

My biggest "Aha!" is that I am facing difficult and hard realities now—I think my preoccupation with my weight was a substitute for dealing with them!

When I look into my heart now, I know my assumptions simply aren't true for me anymore, and I feel like I can no longer go back to the place where I believed them.

Miriam's Biggest Test

Miriam knew the next test she needed to run was with her husband Paul. She also knew this test was going to be the biggest one, the hardest one, the scariest one for her and that she needed to be ready for it. She deliberately took several weeks after her conversation with her father to get ready. As she was planning, she was very pleasantly surprised to see how easy it was to eat healthy meals, to stick to her meditation and yoga practice, and to provide herself with positive feedback about how she was doing. Suddenly, it was all seeming to be much easier than it had ever been before.

People were also starting to notice changes in her. Every day she got comments from friends and colleagues about how happy, healthy, and thin she was looking. "What are you doing?" they all wanted to know. Miriam enjoyed the compliments and felt they made it easier for her to continue giving herself positive reinforcement. But the comments also helped her remain aware of the work she still needed to do. She met with Solange for coffee at least once a week, and together they discussed her plans for her test.

Miriam's Final Test

My Big Assumption Says:	So I will (Change my Behavior This Way)…	And collect the following data …	In Order to Find Out Whether …
I assume that I must keep myself small and limit my potential in order to preserve love and approval in my family.	I will tell Paul that I want to be taking my work more seriously to explore my potential and work toward being a Program Director. I will be honest with him about what that means in terms of additional responsibilities, additional training/education, longer hours, and more travel. Before the conversation, I will have investigated the possibilities for relying on friends, relatives, and other babysitting services to make sure our kids' basic needs can be met when I'm not available for them. Like I did with my dad, I will plan out everything I want to say and imagine some different ways he might respond. I will decide how I would like to respond to him in each of these cases. I will also need to get myself ready, emotionally, for the possibility that he will want a divorce.	What do I say to Paul? What does he say to me? How do I feel (while I'm planning, during the conversation, afterward)? Is there anyone to whom you'd like to give a "heads-up" or ask to serve as an observer who can give you feedback after the fact? Solange is helping me plan, practice, and debrief again. She has been an incredible source of support.	I can make a case for what I truly believe about what I want and communicate this to him. I can bear the possibility that he will disapprove or even reject me completely without caving in on my own truth. I can bear my own feelings of guilt about not being the type of wife/mom that he wants me to be. We can find a way to work out a new type of relationship that allows me to be true to my own deepest wants and needs.

Miriam – Interpretation of Test Data

My Big Assumption says:

I assume that I must keep myself small and limit my potential in order to preserve love and approval in my family.

So in order to test it I changed my behavior this way:

I planned out everything I wanted to say and decided how I would like to respond to Paul in each of these cases. It was difficult to come to terms with the idea that he might want a divorce, but I also knew that I have gotten to a place where there is no going back to who I have been. I couldn't be the same person he married even if I tried. I investigated the possibilities for relying on friends, relatives, and other babysitting services to make sure our kids' basic needs can be met when I'm not available for them.

I told Paul that I want to be taking my work more seriously to explore my potential and work toward being a Program Director. I was very honest with him about what that means in terms of additional responsibilities, additional training/education, longer hours, and more travel. All of that is going to affect the kids and affect him too.

This is what I observed happening:

I didn't get the chance to tell Paul all that I had planned to say though. I got through most of it, but he really couldn't listen because he was pretty upset (pacing around and yelling). But I was prepared for that possibility too. I just sat and listened as long as I could, but I didn't back down. I had used the Difficult Conversations book again, and so I made sure to keep telling him how I felt about him and the kids, as well as how I felt about my work. Finally, he just ended the conversation and went for a drive by himself.

Then Monday night, we talked about it again. He was calmer, and I had a chance to say the rest of the things I had planned. I also tried to ask him a lot of questions about how he was feeling, what his fears were, what was at stake for him. I think that because I knew our whole relationship might likely blow up in my face, I was somehow calmer in this conversation than I have ever been with him. I had accepted that the worst might happen, and so I could focus on just saying my truth and hearing his. I know this must be incredibly hard for him, but I also know it has to be this way for me too. I'm so tired of how things have been.

We didn't really finish talking, and I'm really still not sure what will happen with our marriage. We have a lot to work out.

This is what the data tells me about my Big Assumption:

I can make a case that I truly believe about what I want and communicate it to Paul.

I can bear his disapproval and even the possibility that he will reject me completely. I see now that I am not willing to cave in on my own truth. I am no longer willing to make myself small or limit my potential, even if others resist that.

He did try to make me feel guilty about the kids and about not being the type of wife who will support him and his work the way he wants. That part was the worst. But I can bear the guilt. I did get angry with him for trying to make me feel so bad. And it made me think, "How can he possibly love me when I am not what he wants at all?" He never said "divorce," but I feel like that possibility was always in the room. I guess I learned though that I'm not going to be the one to raise that issue yet. I don't know if he can change. I don't know if we'll stay together. We are for now, I guess.

Your Move

What will your next test be? Use your Change Journal to design and run additional tests, helping you learn more and more about your Big Assumption.

Carla's Tests: Keeping the Weight Off

Carla was a Software Engineer and very good at her job. Often, others she worked with looked to her to teach them something, troubleshoot, or help them out when they ran into a problem. "I feel like I am an enabler. I have a hard time saying no," she explained. Last year, Carla lost a significant amount of weight by paying more attention to diet and exercise. However, as her workload continued to increase, her stress levels also rose, and she was finding it hard to make sure she had enough time to exercise and to be careful about what she ate. She knew she needed to get better at saying "no" to others so that she could make sure she was taking good care of herself.

Here is her ITC map:

Carla

My Improvement Goal	"Doing and Not Doing"	Hidden Completing Commitments	My Big Assumptions
• I am committed to getting better at investing in myself by maintaining my priorities, which means not having to react to whatever comes up, letting others take on more and figure things out for themselves.	• When someone asks for help, I say, "Sure, no problem." I tell them it is easy for me to fix.. • I tend to play down how easy/ hard it was for me to figure it out. • I don't tell my boss or others above her that this is a problem.. • I don't make a big deal of this problem to others.	Worry box: I fear that this will escalate and come back as negative feedback in my report, that the work won't get done (or done right), that I will hurt my colleagues' feelings or make them feel stupid, that if I told my boss the issue will get resolved temporarily but would come back again, that if I don't help I'll be seen as less valuable. • I am committed to not making the situation worse by trying to resist helping them. • I am committed to not being the person who makes someone else feel bad about themselves • I am committed to not having to figure out how to stop that cycle/ pattern. • I am committed to proving my worth, to not being seen as less valuable.	• I assume that I am the only one that can fix it, that they can't. • I assume that if I say "no," the other person will not be able to do it, will do it poorly, or will cause more problems. • I assume that if the other person can't or won't do it, then it will end up creating more work for me to clean up their mess and do it myself. • I assume that if they feel bad about themselves, they wouldn't deal with the situation and would make it an even bigger situation than it is by complaining, etc. • I assume my worth, in others' eyes, is mainly about helping them out.

After creating her Picture of Progress, Carla began observing her BAs. In particular, she noticed "it is always the same people who create the interference" who "always wait until the last minute and then need my help right away."

When one of her colleagues asked for help during a time when Carla had planned to go exercise, she decided to run a spontaneous test. She took three deep breaths before responding. Then she told the colleague she had another appointment. Later, she said, "The three breaths helped. My immediate response was to say yes. I put a note on my desk that said, 'breathe'." At first, it was hard for Carla to enjoy her workout: "When I started the workout, it was hard to get into it. I felt a little bit guilty. I told myself it was OK. And then when I started working out, endorphins kicked in. I was happy later that I had."

In fact, she could see that she had made the right decision. While her colleague was stressed when Carla turned down her request, Carla reasoned, "but it wasn't really an emergency, just an emergency in her mind." She reflected back on her BA and realized "I'm getting to the point where I can tolerate people getting ticked. Maybe that BA isn't as important as I thought." She also saw that her decision may have been "kind of a realization to them that they are dependent on me. Before, I felt like I have to prove my worth by responding right away. What I saw was that by delaying, I could let them see how dependent they are on me."

Carla was ready to run a more ambitious test. At the end of every year, her department had to go back over all their records to track major projects and create spreadsheet records. Usually Carla would just complete this project herself, but she knew it took up too much of her time and that this project was never in her job description. Since she kept very thorough notes about what she had done in past years, she decided she would ask if there was someone else who could use her notes, follow her instructions, and complete the project instead of her.

In fact, the project actually fell under her colleague Amy's job description, but when Carla asked her to take it on, Amy began to offer lots of excuses for why she couldn't. So Carla suggested that Amy do the project with another colleague (Regina) who did seem interested in taking it on. Carla was surprised to notice that she did not feel upset. But she did worry a bit that that the project wouldn't get done, and that she would end up having to do it anyway. Meanwhile, she started tracking the amount of time she was spending helping others when they were stuck. She discovered that the majority of her time was spent with Amy, trying to help her, and if she could just change that pattern, she would make a significant difference in her own schedule.

She decided to talk to Amy about this pattern. After the meeting, Carla reflected on what she had learned. "I think I got a picture into Amy's thinking. She only wants to do what is safe for her. I think everything that is new to her feels unsafe, unless there is someone holding her hand. She's never had to deal with this kind of responsibility before. I don't think she could quickly get to the level where she could deal with this project on her own. I see now that she is looking at my notes on this project as if they are a book written in Greek."

She decided that for the project to work, she might be able to rely more on Regina and think explicitly about how Regina could be helping Amy learn more. After running that test, she wrote about how it had gone:

Carla -- Interpretation of Test Data

My Big Assumption says:

I assume that I am the only one that can fix it or handle something, that they can't.

So in order to test it I changed my behavior this way

I tried to think of a way we could all win, a way to make the project as easy as possible for Amy to learn and take over. I asked Regina if she wanted to try doing it and then also asked Amy to follow along with a copy of the instructions and document any steps that were missing or might be confusing.

This is what I observed happening

They both agreed and I only had to assist when they ran into a very technical issue.

It was a little bit of a struggle for Amy because Regina had to keep prompting her to write down step-by-step directions. Amy kept forgetting to do it, but Regina would stop and get her to do that.

And this is what it tells me about my Big Assumption

This all kind of blew up my Big Assumption. I could see that if I take enough time and figure out how to provide the support for others, they can take on more work than they have.

Her most ambitious, but completely unplanned, test came about a month later when Carla developed a serious virus. "Getting so sick has blown my BA out of the water," she noted. "There were so many things I couldn't do because I would just get so tired. My co-workers have been really good because I needed help even to do the simplest things. I got a little bit of pushback, people telling me 'I don't know how to do that.' But they had to learn how to do it because I couldn't help them. They made some mistakes and got really frustrated at times. But what I have learned is that it is best for me to reassure them, and help them to learn, fix mistakes. It was weird at first, but now I'm enjoying seeing them grow and helping them learn how to troubleshoot. I haven't had any regrets about not being able to help them during my illness because it has been such a strain just getting myself dressed and in to work.

That incident changed everything for Carla, and even after she healed, she thought about her work differently than she had before. She focused less on getting projects done and more on developing people to learn how to take on these projects. "There are still times when I'll hear someone discussing things, and I'll know they are on the wrong path. I could just tell them, but sometimes it is better to have them try and work through it themselves. In those situations, I take three breaths and stop myself before I say anything. I'll ask them to show me what they did instead of me going through and showing them what to do."

While getting sick was obviously unplanned, Carla could clearly see how the work she had been doing on her immunities helped her deal with the situation. "If I had gotten that virus a year ago, I would have been in a total panic that everyone else would be messing things up, and I'd be so worried that all my projects were not going to get done. I would have thought people were not willing to help out, that they couldn't learn. I would have forced myself to do stuff, even if it did compromise my health. Now I am much better at taking care of myself." And getting back to the whole reason she explored this immunity in the first place, she explained, "I make sure I schedule time every day to make a healthy lunch for work. I create a time every day in my schedule for exercise. I make sure I get enough sleep at night. I am maintaining my weight loss!"

All of this learning has made a significant impact on Carla's health. She has found a way to maintain a healthy weight, to exercise regularly to build her strength and flexibility, and to make sure that she makes her own health a priority. She reflected, "The whole process has been so eye-opening. The assumptions that I had have all been blown out of the water. I wouldn't have really believed I could make this big a change back when I started this work, but I guess I have to believe it because I really did it. And I have no fear of going back to how things were before."

10

Taking Stock

The whole process has been incredibly eye-opening. My Big Assumption turned out to be wrong. Period. Now I almost can't believe I used to think that way, that I hadn't seen all this before!

— *Michelle*

If you have run enough tests of your Big Assumptions you should by now be seeing the effects of changing your mind. You are ready then to begin taking stock of what you have done. The work in this chapter is to help you consolidate the new connections you are making between how you think and what you do, between brain and behavior.

We hope that by now you have seen substantial personal progress towards your improvement goal. You may also be wondering whether you are going to be able to sustain your good progress. We all have had experiences of slipping back into old habits and patterns, so we can legitimately ask, "why should it be any different this time?" One way to help yourself not slip back is to consolidate your current progress toward overcoming your immunity. This exercise is designed to help you do just that.

By assessing where you are in a developmental sequence, you will be able to make informed choices about what next steps will deepen your new learning and solidify the bridge you have built. This means testing its foundations, making sure it is well designed and anchored in place, and then traveling across the bridge to see how safe and comfortable you feel. After that, you should be able to cross the bridge whenever you identify a difficult problem or situation you'd like to change. First, let us ask you a few questions. Don't hurry through these. You'll get much more out of this chapter if you set aside thirty minutes or so to engage them. Record your answers in your Change Journal.

Reviewing Your Process and Outcomes

Question 1: Have you reached any conclusions, or noticed any hunches about conditions under which your Big Assumption is *valid*? Think about particular situations – who, what, where and when.

Question 2: Have you reached any conclusions, or noticed any hunches about conditions under which your Big Assumption is *invalid*? Think about particular situations – who, what, where, and when.

Question 3: Do you find your Big Assumption asserting itself in situations where you know it ought not? If so, do you have any generalizations about the conditions under which you are likely (more or less) to find yourself being sucked into the old patterns associated with the Big Assumption? What still sometimes *hooks* you?

Question 4: Are there key "releases" (i.e., ways to get unstuck) you have developed and can use to help yourself easily and readily when you are facing a reappearance of your Big Assumption in real-time?

Question 5: To what extent / how often can you use these "releases" to help you from being back pulled into your old patterns?

Question 6: Have you developed new behaviors or ways of talking to yourself in situations that used to activate your Big Assumption?

Question 7: Think about situations in which you think your Big Assumption is no longer accurate. What new beliefs or understandings do you hold about "how things work" or what will happen in these situations?

Question 8: How would you rate your progress toward achieving your Column 1 goal? Has your understanding of, or relationship to, that goal changed in important ways?

From Where You Are To Where You Want To Be

Let's take a moment to reflect on how far you have come. When you first picked up this book and decided to use it, you were probably ***Unconsciously Immune.*** You may not have known what an immunity to change was, and you didn't know how your own worked. You may not have known how and why you had been unable to lose weight and keep it off. You were immune and you weren't aware of it.

UNCONSCIOUSLY IMMUNE
"I'm completely stuck and I don't know why!"

CONSCIOUSLY IMMUNE:
"I'm still stuck but now I know why and what to do!"

CONSCIOUSLY RELEASED:
"I'm making progress by tending to my immunities mindfully!"

UNCONSCIOUSLY RELEASED:
"I am free of the immunity I worked on and making (or maintaining) progress automatically!"

Revisiting the steps you have taken so far should help you realize that you truly "own" your bridge. First, you created a powerful immunity-to-change map to show you how and why you have had such a hard time maintaining a healthy weight. At that point, you were ***Consciously Immune*** – still stuck, but you knew what to do about it: explore and alter the Big Assumptions that were keeping you stuck in a "safe" place even though you wanted to be somewhere else.

If you've been diligently working through the exercises in this book, you have done that work already. If you are ***Consciously Released*** you are probably learning (through your tests) when your Big Assumption is and is not valid. You may even have discovered that your Big Assumption is inaccurate in most (or all) situations. Often people learn new behaviors and new ways of talking to themselves as a part of this testing process. When you don't rely on your Big Assumption in situations where it is not valid, you are demonstrating the new capacity to be consciously released from it. It may be hard work for you to stop relying on it, and getting to that point usually takes mindful practice. The journey is rarely bump-free or straightforward. It is normal to fall back into old patterns associated with the Big Assumption. Still, knowing that you're falling back, and knowing how you can get yourself unstuck are all signs of progress. You should also see that you have made progress towards meeting your Column 1 goal.
When you no longer need to stop, think, and plan in order to interrupt your Big Assumption, you have developed the capacity to be ***Unconsciously Released*** from it. In situations where your Big Assumption is no longer valid, you automatically act and think in ways that you weren't able to before. New beliefs and understandings, informed and developed mindfully throughout the process, have taken the place of the Big Assumption. You have likely made significant progress, if not full success, towards meeting your improvement goal.

Question 9: Where do you see yourself in the sequence at this time? Record your response in your Change Journal (p. CJ-39)

This stock-taking exercise will be a useful summary of your work to date whether your self-assessment is that you are "Unconsciously Released," or "Consciously Released." Because it usually takes longer than the few months you have presumably been journeying with this book to become "Unconsciously Released," it is more likely that you will see yourself somewhere around "Consciously Released." This means you may want to continue with further tests of your Big Assumption (a good choice especially if you are aware that your Big Assumption grabs hold of you frequently). You can use the results of this exercise to focus those tests. As you run more tests, you will continue to learn more. The new behaviors and ways of thinking you are trying on will become more and more natural to you, and you will continue to move further along toward "Unconsciously Released." Keep testing until you know you are free of your Big Assumption in situations where it is not true. Remember, once you've built your bridge you can cross it as many times as you feel the need.

Ron's Self-Assessment

Improvement Goal: I'm committed to getting better at eating healthier when I'm around other people – at the bar, at parties, at meetings where there is food.

Ron described himself as consciously released. The reason he placed himself there was that he still felt that there were some situations – such as at the bar, at larger family gatherings, and food-related events (such as weddings and some parties) – where he could feel like he wasn't quite a part of things if he was trying to make good choices about what he ate. He wondered if he'd always feel that way. But overall, Ron was thrilled with the progress he had made. "You know," he explained, "maybe I'll always feel a little strange that I can't eat the way I used to. But there are so many problems overeating caused for me too – for my health and my energy and even how I felt about myself. So even if I'm going to feel a little weird sometimes, and even if I feel like I'm always kind of working hard to be healthier, it is absolutely worth it!"

Ron – Self Assessment

What was your Big Assumption?

I assume (no matter what my friends do) that I'll feel less a part of things if I am not eating like my friends are eating.

Where do you see yourself in the sequence at this time?

Consciously released.

Have you reached any conclusions, or developed any hunches about conditions under which your Big Assumption is valid? Think about particular situations – who, what, where and when.

At the bar with the guys
At big parties (like holiday parties and big family gatherings where there is lots of amazing food that everyone is talking about)
Sometimes at restaurants

Have you reached any conclusions, or developed any hunches about conditions under which your Big Assumption is invalid? Think about particular situations – who, what, where, and when.

It is not valid at work anymore. Everyone there knows I've changed, and they are only trying to help. In my day-to-day life, it doesn't usually come up, which is great!

Do you find your Big Assumption asserting itself in situations you know it ought not? If so, do you have any generalizations about the conditions under which you are likely (more or less) to find yourself being sucked into the old patterns associated with the Big Assumption? What still sometimes hooks you?

Sometimes I still do overeat, especially if I'm drinking.

Are there key "releases" (i.e., self-talk that unhooks you) you have developed and can use to help yourself easily and readily when you are facing your Big Assumption in real-time?

I don't spend as much time at the bar, and I don't even go there every week anymore. So even if I do fall off the wagon there, it doesn't really end up becoming too big a problem.

To what extent / how often can you use these "releases" to help you from being pulled into old patterns?

So far, so good.

Have you developed new behaviors or ways of talking to yourself in situations that used to activate your Big Assumption?

I know that it may feel good in the moment that I am eating something or drinking, but I also know that I will not feel good about that later. I have arranged other ways to hang out with the guys (like playing basketball) so we don't spend as much time at the bar. I have other ways of thinking about what "the full experience" even means. I might "miss out" a little on some kinds of things, but I'm getting a lot more out of things that didn't even exist before. I pay more attention to the conversations I have. In some ways, I may feel even closer to some of the guys as a result.

Think about situations in which you think your Big Assumption is no longer accurate. What new beliefs or understandings do you hold about "how things work" or what will happen in these situations?

People do like me, not because of what I eat and drink, and if you want to make a change, they will support you. Usually, I don't feel less a part of things or like I'm missing out. And when I do feel that way, it's not so bad – I can deal with it.

How would you rate your progress toward achieving your Column 1 goal? Has your understanding of or relationship to that goal changed in important ways?

Other people don't make me eat anything. It's all up to me. I have lost about 35 pounds, and I'm not thin, but my doc says that my BP and cholesterol numbers are much better now. I can really feel it too. I feel younger and more energetic. I also feel like I had this monkey on my back for so long because I couldn't see my way out. Now I have a different way of looking at myself – like I can figure out what I need to do!

Miriam's Self-Assessment

Improvement Goal: I'm committed to getting better at creating and following new lifelong food habits – no fad diets, no drastic approaches that I can't keep up.

Miriam had come a long way since she had first created her immunity map. She was amazed at how well she had been able to develop and follow new lifelong eating and exercise habits. And she was amazed that in the process of working on this goal, she had completely transformed the rest of her life as well. By the time she was ready to take stock of where she had come in this long process, Miriam felt as though she had become "a different person."

"Some of the Big Assumptions I had when I created my map are just no longer true. I don't believe there is anything wrong with me. I think what was wrong was that I was afraid to be honest with myself about what would really make me happy. I was afraid to listen to my heart because I knew it could make other people angry at me, and I feared their judgment. But once I really came to terms with my own goals, I also knew that I couldn't keep sacrificing them. Even if that made people angry with me. I am not worthless. I learned I actually have quite a lot to offer – to myself, to my family, and to the world. So I feel unconsciously released from my BA that if I don't criticize myself really harshly, I'll slack off too much."

In the process of learning about that Big Assumption, I also have learned about my other Big Assumptions and I feel unconsciously released from them as well:

- I assume that if I try to lose weight, I will actually feel worse, be under more pressure, and I will fail.
- I assume I have even bigger faults than my weight that will keep me unhappy, and if I get thin I will have to face these, and I won't be able to deal with them.

Miriam felt like she was still learning about the three new assumptions that she uncovered while exploring her original one:

- I assume that I must keep myself small and limit my potential in order to preserve love and approval in my family.
- I assume that if I don't criticize myself, others will.
- I assume if people saw the real me, they would reject me.

She had learned that important relationships in her family – such as her relationship with her father – were not based on keeping herself small or hiding who she really was. "My dad may be angry. He may be disappointed. But he still loves me. And what I learned was, that is enough. I had assumed that I needed his approval. I had assumed that approval and love were the same thing. But they are not. My dad can love me and will love me even if my own path is different than what he wanted for me." As Miriam talked with other members of her family, this key realization was further reinforced and helped her identify a final assumption she had been working on throughout, "I assume that I must have their approval if they are to love me and I am to love myself." And she knew that assumption no longer felt true.

Miriam also reflected on how the changes in her life had affected her marriage. "Well, that's a work in progress, but I am no longer expecting to be separated anytime soon," she explained. "We've all had growing pains. Paul, the kids, and me. And we're still learning how we're going to be the best family we can be for each other. So that's hard." She paused and smiled. "But it is good too. I got my promotion, and by the time I finally got the courage to ask for it, I knew that I absolutely deserved it."

She continued, "And even though I think Paul misses the good old days when I was more the type of wife he had in mind, I think he has also appreciated some of the new changes too. I'm happier. I have more energy. I definitely look and feel much better. And I love, love, love my work. So when I am home, which is not as much as he'd like, I know, I love being there too. I'm so happy to see everyone. I'm so happy to be a wife and a mother and to feel like I'm doing the best damn job with my life that I can." Miriam suddenly laughed. "Oh yeah, and with my promotion, we have more money now too, which is a pretty good thing as well!"

"I can't tell you how great I feel to have my eating habits under control. I mean, that was my original goal. That's what started this whole transformation in the first place." She decided to take stock of the three assumptions that she hadn't completely rejected already.

Miriam – Self Assessment

What was your Big Assumption?

I assume that I must keep myself small and limit my potential in order to preserve love and approval in my family.
I assume that if I don't criticize myself, others will.
I assume if people saw the real me, they would reject me.

Where do you see yourself in the sequence at this time?

Consciously released on these I think. With every step I have taken, I have become clearer about what I want and need. And I see that I need to be true to myself no matter what.

Have you reached any conclusions, or developed any hunches about conditions under which your Big Assumption is valid? Think about particular situations – who, what, where and when.

People may not approve of what I do. And they may even decide to reject me because of the choices I have made. So I guess that part can be valid, although I guess none of that seems to matter as much as it did before.

Have you reached any conclusions, or developed any hunches about conditions under which your Big Assumption is invalid? Think about particular situations – who, what, where, and when.

The big thing that is different is that I used to feel like I couldn't deal with someone rejecting me. I thought that I needed their approval for me to love myself! Now I know I have to do what is in my heart, even if that means others will be disappointed, even if they are so disappointed that they won't want to be with me.

Do you find your Big Assumption asserting itself in situations you know it ought not? If so, do you have any generalizations about the conditions under which you are likely (more or less) to find yourself being sucked into the old patterns associated with the Big Assumption? What still sometimes hooks you?

I still can feel guilty if I haven't seen the kids in a while and I am not there to go to all their concerts and sports events. Often, I'm not the first one they tell about their bad day at school — or their good day at school either. There are many times when I feel such regret about that.

Are there key "releases" (i.e., self-talk that unhooks you) you have developed and can use to help yourself easily and readily when you are facing your Big Assumption in real-time?

The thing that I tell myself that always brings me back to good feelings again is how much happier I am now. And in the end, I guess I believe that actually makes me a better mom. I never thought of myself as a role model for them before, but now I do. Now I think, "that's right, kids. You need to follow your dreams. You need to make your life work for you." I hope they are learning that from me. I hope they can see just how amazing my life feels now. I think they can. The other day my daughter asked me, "How come you are so happy lately?" So, she sees how I've changed. She sees that.

To what extent / how often can you use these "releases" to help you from being pulled into old patterns?

Well, eating and exercise and yoga have only gotten easier. I mean my schedule is much crazier, but I really don't fall of the wagon much at all. It has gotten to the point where I really can't figure out why that all used to be so hard in the first place!

Have you developed new behaviors or ways of talking to yourself in situations that used to activate your Big Assumption?

Seeing myself as a role model for my kids is one. And making sure I continue to work on my marriage is another. We both are working hard to communicate better with each other and to not "keep score" about how we can disappoint each other.

Think about situations in which you think your Big Assumption is no longer accurate. What new beliefs or understandings do you hold about "how things work" or what will happen in these situations?

I believe people can change. I did. Paul did, even though he didn't want to. Seeing that has made me such a believer in going after my goals and really stretching myself to find out what I am capable of becoming. People ask me all the time how I lost the weight, and boy, that's a long story. But I always look them straight in the eye and tell them, "I had to start on the inside. I had to figure out who I really was and wasn't." I don't know if that is the answer they want, but that's the truth.

How would you rate your progress toward achieving your Column 1 goal? Has your understanding of or relationship to that goal changed in important ways?

I have lost 50 pounds, and I have stayed at that weight for a few months now. Time will tell if I have lost all I can lose, or if I can still lose a few more. More importantly, I feel like I have a whole new life. I didn't know that is what I was really working on when all this began!!

Glenn's Self-Assessment

Before I started this ITC process, I ate too much and drank too much. I smoked too. And I was a pretty heavy drinker. Alcohol was a release from any day-to-day discomforts or annoyances I was facing. I even experimented with drugs, although luckily, I never liked them. But alcohol slowed my mind down and helped me avoid feeling anything unpleasant. I quit drinking a while before I ever heard about ITC. I was proud of that, but it had come at a cost. Once I quit drinking, food very quickly became my favorite strategy for avoiding my feelings.

My father was always very authoritarian with me – very quick to criticize and tell me what to do. The best strategy was always just to obey and stay out of his way. My parents separated when I was a sophomore in high school. They had a terrible relationship and were always fighting, so maybe the divorce was a good thing, but I was very upset about it. I learned how to handle this situation with the very things that appear in my third column as hidden commitments:

- I am committed to being safe, to not being hurt.
- I am committed to not feeling out of control.
- I am committed to not being rejected or cast aside.
- I am committed to avoiding conflict.
- I am committed to not feeling my feelings.

I could see very quickly that my BA was:

"If I stop eating so much I will have to feel my feelings – feel the terrible awareness that I may not be very safe, in control, or accepted. I will be more aware of the potential for conflict and for being hurt, rejected, or cast aside."

It hit me like a ton of bricks. I had internalized my father's punishing voice.

I assumed that I had to be so critical with myself because I believed that would keep me 'in line' – in other words, safe, in control, accepted."

Seeing my immune system was incredibly freeing because I could look at it and name it. All of a sudden I could see that I had a choice. I had done therapy for about five years, and it was very helpful to me in other respects. So I had done a lot of self-exploration. But it is amazing to me how, in a one-hour session creating my immunity map, I could name something I had never been able to see in therapy. I could see that my immunity had been pulling me to behave in a certain way, driving me more than I was driving it. And all of a sudden, it was like, 'I can now choose to drive. I can choose to let these things have power or authority over me, or I can choose to change them.'"

Once I did the map, I started saying "f--- you" to that voice that was holding me back. I knew if I needed to go to the next level, I was going to have to be a little unsafe, lose a little control. My first test was to talk to my wife, to tell her what I had found out in my map. When I told her about my assumptions that I would be rejected and cast aside, she looked me right in the eyes and said, 'That's crazy, Glenn.' That was all I needed. I sort of knew that was true, but still, it was like the old me kept holding me back. So I ran more tests. I would dip my toes in, challenge the BAs to see what happened.

Five years ago I weighed 226 pounds, but now I've been at about 170 for the past three years. Even when I first started losing weight through ITC I was still being very, very hard on myself. Very rigid. But over time, I began to gain much more confidence, and I realized that the negative self-talk was limiting me. I think I eventually realized through this work that I needed to learn how to forgive myself. I can still notice that I'll shift into self-criticism very quickly. So I guess I'm still observing myself. And sometimes my wife catches me too. I just remind myself that these stories are all in my head, and I can write whatever I want.

As my context has changed, my challenges in keeping the weight off have changed. I'll see some final remnants of my BAs show up occasionally in new and different ways. Becoming a parent introduced a whole host of new things, and in general, I feel like I have had to get used to having less control, less time, less energy. Right now we have little goldfish crackers all over the house.

I had to get more creative about how to make sure I exercise and to make sure it is a priority. When I am not creative I get stuck in the rules that I had created for myself – like I will tell myself I need to find a 60-minute block of time to exercise, or that I need to go to the gym to get a good workout in. Well, that's not going to happen as easily anymore, so I need to challenge myself to rethink. I see that I was making up rules that aren't necessarily there. My wife and I walk every morning, and I keep a treadmill in my office for when I can find ten or twenty minutes here and there.

This whole journey has been hard to talk about and describe. But lots of people wanted to know what I did to lose all the weight. The first time I told the whole story out loud, I cried hard. I think I've never cried that hard before. There was something in me that was released. That was another step toward letting go of the way I had been before.

Glenn – Self Assessment

Where do you see yourself in the sequence at this time?

Somewhere between Consciously Released and Unconsciously Released.

Have you reached any conclusions, or developed any hunches about conditions under which your Big Assumption is *valid*? Think about particular situations – who, what, where and when.

They are not true at all. Being hard on myself wasn't really helping anybody, although maybe it did keep me out of my father's way. But I remember the boy I was when I was 4, before things between my parents got bad. I was just being myself then, just very unselfconscious. I feel like the last several years have been a journey back to finding that little boy who I was.

Have you reached any conclusions, or developed any hunches about conditions under which your Big Assumption is *invalid*? Think about particular situations – who, what, where, and when.

It is not valid in any circumstances of my life right now. Not only have I lost weight, I've also made other breakthroughs – conquering my fear of public speaking for example. I'm much more confident about anything new I'm trying to learn.

Do you find your Big Assumption asserting itself in situations you know it ought not? If so, do you have any generalizations about the conditions under which you are likely (more or less) to find yourself being sucked into the old patterns associated with the Big Assumption? What still sometimes hooks you?

I can't think of anything that is hooking me right now. But when my circumstances change dramatically, as they did when I became a father, it might come up again in some new way I haven't had to face yet. I am not sure if I could really get hooked by it again though, because I am so aware of it and have done so much work. It has little power anymore, even if I can't say for certain that it has gone away completely.

Are there key "releases" (i.e., self-talk that unhooks you) you have developed and can use to help yourself easily and readily when you are facing your Big Assumption in real-time?

Many. Self-talk is a big one. Saying "f--- you" to it was the first one I found that worked. I have found for me that it is always good to get angry at something as a way to make it less a part of me, make it have less power over me. In general, I just watch my thinking much more than I ever did before. I just watch it, and sometimes negative thoughts just fade away when I name them for what they are.

To what extent / how often can you use these "releases" to help you from being pulled into old patterns?

All the time right now.

Have you developed new behaviors or ways of talking to yourself in situations that used to activate your Big Assumption?

See Above.

Think about situations in which you think your Big Assumption is no longer accurate. What new beliefs or understandings do you hold about "how things work" or what will happen in these situations?

I feel like I am very aware of how much possibility there is in any situation. If I start to think something is hard, or unlikely, or bad for me, I almost immediately also start to generate ideas for how it could work. I see myself as having unlimited potential.

How would you rate your progress toward achieving your Column 1 goal? Has your understanding of or relationship to that goal changed in important ways?

I am pretty happy at 170. The lowest I got down to was 168. I am thinking that I might want to try to cut back more on carbs – cut out gluten completely – and see what kind of effect that has on how I feel. I've heard it is common to lose a few pounds from cutting that out, which would be fine, but that's not really what is motivating me so much now.

The Journey Never Ends

It is not uncommon for our clients to feel like their stock-taking brings their official ITC work to a close, even if they continue to run tests and keep making self-observations in informal ways. For others, taking stock helps them identify places where they might still feel stuck and so leads them to design and run new tests in those areas. This can be a great time to go back and take a look at your Picture of Progress. When do you see yourself if that progression? Should some of those doing/thinking/feeling descriptors be re-written now that you are clearer what "Significant Progress" actually looks like?

It is also not uncommon for clients to feel that in overturning one immunity in their life, they are ready to use this approach again, turning their attention to a new goal.

For example, once Ron succeeded in losing weight and getting in better shape, his new goal became "keeping the weight off," and he started the ITC process all over again. You'll see his new map in the next chapter.

CONCLUSION

Owning Your Bridge

This process is very deep. It is not a Sunday afternoon project.

— Ula

Now I am in a position where I cannot justify not going for anything I want. I have begun asking myself, "what would I do if I knew I couldn't fail?" This process accelerates following your inner compass. It is a fantastic tool to go about this in a conscious way and make it happen much faster.

— Tomas

In most cases, if you told the authors of a book that you "couldn't put it down," that you read it from cover to cover in a few days, they would be happy and flattered.

But we wouldn't.

We weren't trying to transport you to another world the way great fiction can, or to stimulate your mind alone with a set of new ideas. On the contrary, we were trying to bring you closer in to the real world you are living in today, to *apply* a set of ideas—so that you live in your world with the greater satisfaction of accomplishing a goal that has been as elusive for you as it has been important.

Specifically, we wrote it so you could be *lighter*. Lighter in body *weight*, yes; but you want to *stay* lighter — and that can only happen by becoming lighter in *mind*, as well. Right Weight/Right Mind.

We wrote this book to help you *offload*—not just the pounds or kilos—but those constraining Big Assumptions you may not even have known you were carrying around, day after day, week after week, year after year. They have been weighing you down. They are the source of the pervasive "ordinary suffering" we have been witness to, the resignation and self-contempt that sets in from repeatedly failing at personal change goals despite our smartest plans, our most heartfelt intentions, and our most strenuous and sincere efforts.

We are crossing our fingers that you didn't just read this book through in a couple of sittings, so let's imagine together for a moment what the experience would be of someone who did. At the best, he or she might have learned some new ideas about what prevents us from changing, or making changes that last. By reading the stories and examples she or he might even see these ideas "come to life" enough to do a passable job explaining to someone what the book is about.

These readers might know now what "the immunity to change" is, but there is no chance they are going to succeed with their improvement goals because they haven't really explored *their own* immunities to change, and they haven't done the work involved in offloading them.

If you *have* actually done that work on your own immunity it should now be many weeks since you first picked this book up, and you have put it down, many, many times. You put it down to engage in the set of practices and exercises we offered you. You put it down to do things, *things* in your head and things out in your world. We congratulate you for doing all that hard work, and getting to this point!

We want to use this Conclusion to help you get even more out of the hard work you have done. We will first invite you to step back a bit from your hard work and take a look at it, to make sure you see what you have actually done, what you have actually *built*. We think this will increase the chances that you will see the book was not just an itinerary for a single trip. In taking your journey in this original way you have really created a new kind of vehicle you can use to reach *any* destination that has proven difficult to get to (or difficult to stay there once you have first arrived).

The Idea of the Bridge

What have you actually done? The exercises have gotten you into the *particulars* of your own *unique* Big Assumptions. You are, at best, only a few months into working on a new relationship, not to "Big Assumptions" as an abstract category, but to your *particular* self-limiting beliefs. So it would be completely understandable if you did not yet fully appreciate that what we have been helping you develop can be useful to you in many other ways.

You haven't been reading and working with this book all by yourself. Thousands of others have been going through the same exercises you have, working on getting free from *completely different* beliefs, perhaps, but those of you who have succeeded with these tools have all developed the same new strengths. You have all built the identical thing. What is it?

We have talked throughout the book about a "bridge" that wasn't there for you when you began reading this book. There are many ways to see this bridge, and to talk about it. We can do so quite metaphorically, but we can also root it in the two well-researched sciences of the mind and of the brain.

At the simplest level, when it comes to accomplishing personal change goals, like those around eating and fitness, people have a clear (and often agonized) sense of Where I Am, and a (hopeful or despairing) sense of Where I Want to Be. What they lack is a sense of a trustworthy bridge that enables them to cross from one side to the other. They may become intrigued with a new fad diet or procedure they think will get them there, but then the bridge collapses before they have crossed over. Or it seems like the bridge has gotten them there, only to discover that it comes with an invisible "rubber band," and before you have spent much time on the other side you are pulled back over the bridge to the place you began.

If you are beginning now to feel some freedom from some of your Big Assumptions (the sort of thing you heard people say in the later chapters, such as "that just seems silly now," or "there is almost no situation where I any longer believe that is true"), it is important that you see you are not just freer of *that particular assumption*. You have built the *vehicle* by which you can get freer of other assumptions as well—not automatically; you still have to do the work and you still have to cross over the bridge again. But the point is, *there is a bridge now*, and it doesn't have a rubber band, or a big toll booth, and you can cross over it any time you want.

How did you do this? Basically, we helped you see that the picture you were creating in your mind of how the world works was not 100% accurate. Instead of just looking through the camera lens of your mind to take pictures, you needed to make some important alterations to your camera lens so that it would take better pictures. At the same time, you were making some new connections among the parts of your camera lens so that these parts are working well together and not causing friction. These processes are explored and explained more fully in two important research communities – that of developmental psychology (the science of the mind) and that of neuroscience (the science of the brain). We're going to briefly layout the fundamentals of these ideas here, for those of you, like us, who find such things fascinating. However, if it bores you to tears, feel free to just skip on to the next section about exploring the width and length of your bridge.

The central idea from the science of the *mind* is that our mind develops (enabling us to see more deeply into ourselves and our world) through our gradual and successive ability to step back and *look* at the lenses we were formerly *looking through*. When we are choicelessly, unmindfully looking at ourselves and the world through a particular lens (thinking what we are really seeing is "the world" and "ourselves" when it is just the world and ourselves *as this lens renders them*) then we could say the lens "has us" (we are captive to it). But when we can *look* at our own lens, make choices about whether we want to see things through that lens, then the lens has become more of a "tool," something "we have." When we overturn our immunities we make this type of shift – to our hidden commitments and to our Big Assumptions.

When your self-protective commitment (e.g., "I am committed to never feeling bored or unstimulated") creates unwanted behaviors (e.g., frequent snacking) often without your even realizing why, that self-protective commitment "has you." When you make the commitment itself less hidden, and begin to examine its source, you begin to "have it," and there is more of a chance you can do something about it. The exercises you have been doing help you move your self-protective commitments from a place where they have you to a place where you have them. This starts the construction of your bridge. You still can't cross it, but it's a start.

When your self-limiting belief (e.g., "if I get thinner it will throw my wife into a tailspin") is narrowing your options without your even realizing it, this mere assumption has become what we call a Big Assumption (an assumption taken unquestioningly, unmindfully as true). It has you. But when you identify it as such, consider it may or may not be true, and give the world a chance to show you whether you should modify it, then you start to "have it" and you begin to build more layers on your bridge.

Your whole immunity to change then starts to become something "you have," rather than it "having you." As you, more and more, are "working on it" rather than it "working on you," you are creating a more and more robust, reliable bridge for crossing over from **Where I Am** to **Where I Want to Be**. **Where I Want to Be** becomes less and less a place of mere hope ("maybe this cleansing thing will finally do it"), or dispiriting despair ("I'll never get there"), or bewildering scam ("I thought I got there, but now I'm back where I started").

Nerdy academicians that we are, we can't resist letting you know that in our terms, the work you have been doing to help strengthen this mind-shift in your way of knowing has been all about helping you move aspects of your thinking and feeling from a place where you are *subject to* them (they run you) to a place where they become an *object* for you (you can make choices about them). This subject-object structure is the very root of our epistemologies, the *ways* we know. One way of understanding the bridge you have built is to see that it starts with the well-anchored pillars on either side of "subject" and "object."

The central idea we are taking from the science of the brain is that there are different parts of the brain performing very different kinds of jobs, and that we are much more effective when they are not working too independently of each other, or at cross purposes.

In particular, the neo-cortex is the seat of judgment, the place where we can analyze and reflect, the place that develops the greater complexity and insight we were just talking about in reference to the mind. The amygdala, a prehistoric inheritance, performs a very important function too. It is continuously scanning the world for possible danger and when it goes into Red Alert it overrides the neo-cortex and other brain functions as well.

The amygdala is the part of the brain we have been referring to as your big, faithful dog that barks ferociously whenever anyone—*anyone!*—approaches the house. If you immediately grab a rifle without thinking and start shooting out the window whenever your dog starts to bark then your dog is running you. As ridiculous a picture as that presents, the humbling evidence from brain science is that that is exactly what we are doing most of the time in the face of threats the amygdala perceives. We don't always "shoot"; that would be the automatic "fight" response. Sometimes we "flee"; we just as automatically withdraw—

physically, or more often emotionally and intellectually. This can be very subtle; we feel a lack of energy, bored, even slightly depressed. The key point though is the "without thinking about it." The neo-cortex is over-ridden and we automatically lose a connection to the more thoughtful, reflective side of ourselves.

Diagnosing and overturning our immunities to change helps us establish these connections:

- When we let the amygdala persist in its overriding of the neo-cortex, there is no bridge between the two.
- When we do not ignore our "barking dog" but don't let it take over either, when we recover from that first burst of adrenaline and alarm and decide to take a look for ourselves out the window before picking up the gun, then we "have the dog" rather than the dog having us.
- When we can do this more regularly, especially around a particular imagined threat (e.g., my spouse going into a tailspin if I lose weight) then we have further built the bridge (with respect to this issue) that will help us cross over from **Where I Am** to **Where I Want to Be**.

The exercises you have been trying on in this book are as rooted in brain science as the science of the developing mind. A cutting-edge area of brain research today called "reconsolidation" (using rats as subjects) deals exactly with the possibility of taking brain activity that has been living in the amygdala (where it cannot come under the governance of the neo-cortex) and moving it into the neo-cortex where it can be modified. "Reconsolidation" is really about "bridge-building" in just the way we have been talking about it, and, in a general sense, the work you have been doing with this book is helping you strengthen your bridge through a kind of "reconsolidation."

You can see this most vividly in the third column of your ITC map and what happens in moving from the Worry Box to the Hidden Commitments. What you are trying to capture in your Worry Box is as close to the activity of the amygdala as possible. We ask you, in imagining your doing the opposite of the behaviors in your second column, *what would be most disturbing* about that (e.g., you listed, in the second column, "I don't eat proper portions. I just keep eating what is on the plate"). If you really vicariously placed yourself in the position of *setting aside* half the serving, or *eating no more* even though you are enjoying the food, your amygdala should be sounding all kinds of alarms ("Oh no, I will be unhappy!" or "Help! I will feel trapped and controlled." Or "Grrr, that is just like my mother taking away my cookies"). These are the feelings you are trying to capture in your Worry Box. They are automatic; there is no way to prevent them, and you don't need to in order not to be run by them.

When we next invite you to reframe these raw worries as "commitments" ("I am committed to never again feeling like I am in 'food jail' and my mother is the warden") we are helping you connect—build a bridge between—your amygdala and your neo-cortex. The raw anger that first came up is the province of the amygdala. Once we convert this into something more abstract like a *motive*, or *intention*, or *commitment*, we have reconsolidated it into the province of the neo-cortex, and, as you hopefully have experienced, this opens up a whole new vista of possibilities for change. That vista comes into view because you have gotten up onto a reliable new bridge.

Exploring the Width and Length of Your Bridge

Now that you have a better understanding of what you have created—the bridge itself—we want to make sure you do not shortchange yourself, and take full advantage of its width and length.

As you have made progress with this book, have you had any thoughts or experiences even a little like this?

> "My ITC map, and my exploration of my Big Assumptions, are definitely helping me with my Column 1 improvement goal, but this is turning out to be about a lot more than food and diet."

This is something we hear a lot, and it is a reflection of the potential "width" of the bridge you built. You may remember Clyde in Chapter 8, the fellow who was concerned about his wife, Bev, possibly going into a depression if he lost weight, or in particular, her being upset if he went off on an exercise run without her after she decided as usual that she didn't want to go. Here is an excerpt from an e-mail he wrote one of us, many months after we had stopped working with him:

> I want to thank you for the way the approach has helped me take off, and keep off, the weight I wanted to lose. But, as I was thinking about all that I learned, I wanted to pass on a much bigger kind of thanks, because this has really gone way beyond diet and way beyond just my relationship with Bev.
>
> My fear about people possibly getting upset, I now realize is a huge life-theme. It has been around forever, and once I started to see how it works with Bev, I began to see it everywhere—at work, with friends, with the guy who repairs my car, for God's sake. What has been most liberating is not just that they rarely are upset or will get upset, it's that I don't automatically think it's necessarily my fault, my responsibility, even my problem, if they do! This has been a real life-changer.

> I learned the Big Danger I had been protecting myself from was not really that someone would be "mad at me." It was more about *what I would do to myself* if they were! I would end up feeling so bad or guilty, beat myself up. I don't do that so much anymore. The dog still barks. I get alarmed for a moment when I think they are going to be upset with me, and I start beating myself up. But then I step in and stop it. "Is this their thing or mine?" I ask myself. The best thing of all is really coming to see that the *sense* of danger is not the same thing as a *real* threat. One doesn't have to mean the other. I'm not sure I ever made this distinction before.

Sometimes people do not take the full advantage of the width of their bridge because they are so focused on the food-related improvement goal. You may find it useful to ask yourself,

- "Have I derived all the possible learnings—and beneficial changes—from my current ITC map?"
- "If I look at the Big Assumptions that no longer have such a grip on me, have they been holding me back in other areas of my life? Can I now consider seeing and behaving differently in these other areas?"
- [If you don't have immediate answers to the prior question:] "Would it be useful for me to re-do the Observations exercise—with respect to those assumptions that no longer feel right—but this time be looking for the way they influence me in other areas of my life?"
- "What about other Big Assumptions in my ITC map that I didn't end up testing [probably because you were able to make progress on your food-related improvement goal without pursuing these]? Might there be benefits in other parts of my life by testing these, now that I've gone to the trouble of surfacing them?"

If there is more to be derived from further exploring your current ITC map, there are even bigger possibilities in *future* maps. You didn't just learn how to create your current map. In the process, you learned a set of practices that can help you bridge from **Where You Are** to **Where You Want to Be** for a host of other improvement goals. This speaks to the *length* of your bridge. We have learned it can span across a myriad of aspirations. Nearly any improvement goal that does not yield to a straight-ahead, incrementally advancing, behavior-change focused, "technical" approach is a candidate for ITC.

Your next map might stay connected to your goals around weight but involve the next challenge after you have taken it off—namely, *keeping* if off. Your immunity to change around keeping it off may implicate a different set of Hidden Commitments and Big Assumptions. For example, once Ron succeeded in losing weight and getting in better shape, he noticed a tendency to tell himself he could ease up. He started weighing himself less frequently (which for him had been helpful; we are not saying everyone needs to weigh themselves regularly). He began to find excuses for not exercising. He decided to create a new map and start the ITC process all over again, this time more tightly focused on the issues surrounding maintenance vs. regaining. The map interested him because some of the third and fourth column themes were different. He enjoyed working his way through the activities again (he didn't do all of them this time), and most importantly, he found that it helped him stay in shape and not regain the weight he had taken off.

Ron

My Improvement Goal	"Doing and Not Doing"	Hidden Counter-Commitments	My Big Assumptions
• I'm committed to maintaining my new healthy lifestyle (better eating and better exercise)	• I tell myself I can ease up more than I used to. • I don't weigh myself regularly, especially when I have eaten more than I should. • I find excuses to not exercise daily.	Worry box: I fear being an annoying fanatic. I fear getting bored or being boring as a one-trick pony. I loathe the idea of becoming a robot, of losing my spontaneity. • I am committed to not being seen as only about my health and weight, and to not feeling myself that I am becoming a fanatic. • I am committed to not losing a relaxed, spontaneous, fun way of being--in life and with others; to not becoming a robot, or mechanical slave to my regimen.	• I assume that if I maintain my new healthy lifestyle, others are going to start to find me annoying; I am going to feel like this is too big a way that people now see me; I am going to feel like I have become a fanatic; I am going to be less spontaneous and fun. • I assume that keeping my new lifestyle will always feel like a bit of an ordeal; that how it feels now is the way it will always feel. • I assume it is black or white; I'm either all in or I become a fat slob again.

Or your next map might stay in the world of health and fitness but take up a completely different kind of issue. For example, many people have difficulty complying with medical advice despite their genuine desire to do so. Heart doctors say they can warn their patients about the life-and-death risks, not just of being overweight, but refusing to take their meds as prescribed, not exercising, smoking, or heavy drinking, and still only about one in seven can actually make these changes. And the other six want to keep living; they literally cannot change to save their own lives.

We have been studying a piece of this problem—patient non-compliance with maintenance medications. Many millions of people are prescribed drugs they should take regularly, perhaps for the rest of their lives. It is carefully explained to them they could, for example, have a stroke and die if they don't regularly take a medicine that will have no negative side effects and is covered by their insurance. They express every intention to follow their doctor's orders, they understand how important it is that they do so, and, still, several studies show that one year later more than half are not compliant.

We have studied people who are baffled by their own inability to regularly take a medication they know they need, and we have been discovering interesting Hidden Commitments and Big Assumptions, previously unknown to the medical world and to the patients themselves, that make their non-compliant behaviors perfectly sensible, even brilliant. For example, Ed is a 50-year old man prescribed three such "maintenance medications." He understands the necessity that he takes them, keenly wants to be compliant, but is not. When he is asked why he isn't, given his wish to be, he really has no good answer. But when he completed his ITC map he understood why, and so will you:

Ed

My Improvement Goal	"Doing and Not Doing"	Hidden Counter-Commitments	My Big Assumptions
• I'm committed to being better at complying with doctor's orders—in particular, being more compliant regarding my medications.	• I don't take them every day as prescribed. • I don't refill them promptly when they run out. • When I get those reminder messages on my voice-mail from the drugstore I just hang up in the middle of the call.	Worry box: Feels like being at death's door; like I am some very old, over-the-hill guy who has to take a drug every day! Like some guy on life-support. • I am committed to not feeling like an old, sick, decrepit, over-the-hill guy, living on life support! • I am committed to not feeling dependent on anyone or anything. • I am committed to not feeling pitiful.	• I assume that anyone who has to take a drug every day is very sick, and pitiful. • I assume having to take a drug every day means you are giving up your independence.

Or perhaps the improvement goal that is now feeling most important and elusive is the one that keeping your job depends upon. As we said in the introduction, we have helped thousands of people identify, and overturn, their immunities to making changes in the ways they operate at work. Now that you have built your bridge its length can extend as far as you like, is there something that keeps coming up on your end-of-year evaluations, something you've tried to get better at that doesn't yield to smart strategies and strenuous efforts? Chances are there is a piece of the picture you are missing.

Consider Annemarie, a star performer with clients in a professional services firm, who nonetheless was told she would need to be let go if she couldn't get on better with her teams. Junior colleagues regularly gave her poor scores and asked not to work with her again. They found her overly critical and micromanaging. Annemarie didn't want to be either of these things, but try as she might, the same self-sabotaging behavior persisted—until she developed a good ITC map, and took the time to test some of her Big Assumptions.

Anne Marie

My Improvement Goal	"Doing and Not Doing"	Hidden Counter-Commitments	My Big Assumptions
• Better team leader—specifically, more supportive and better delegator with junior colleagues.	• Always looking for how their work can be better, much more likely to 'constructively criticize' than praise. • Assign them projects and then over-prescribe how they should go about it, or even take it back sometimes. • Take up a lot of the limelight, be the public face of the team.	Worry box: Being phony, superficial, 'you're great'; they slack off if not always a little nervous; becoming less relevant, more dispensable; preparing my successor and putting myself out of a job. • I am committed to: Not being a glad-handing phony who is always telling people how great they are. • Keeping my people on their back feet, always a little under stress. • Not becoming marginal, being in-dispensable, the most important person on the team. • Not becoming irrelevant. • Not creating my own competition and hastening my replacement.	• I assume praising is a kind of weakness. • I assume people do better under pressure. • I assume the better my people get the less good it is for me (they need me less; others see they can do without me). • I assume my position is securer the more central I am to my team ("I know this one is ridiculous, but there you have it!"). • I assume my greatest value to the team is to "lead from the front."

Afterword

Finally, before we let you go, we want to make sure you understand that your bridge may not only be wider than you have been considering and longer than you have been considering, but also less solitary. Thousands of people now, all over the world, from all walks of life, have built the same basic bridge that you have. Each person's particulars will be unique, of course, but the fundamental work of shifting our thinking from a place where it is running us to a place where we are running it, is common to everyone's experience.

If you'd like to read more about the immunity to change, the theory that underlies it, its applications in work environments, and its in use diagnosing and overturning "team immunities" or other collective immunities: R. Kegan and L. Lahey, *Immunity to Change* (Boston: Harvard Business Press, 2001).

CHANGE JOURNAL

Overcoming the Immunity to Change

This is a purpose-driven journal intended to accompany you as you read *Right Weight/ Right Mind.* We don't just want you to ***read*** the book; we want you to ***do*** the work that will help you overturn your immunities! The biggest purpose of the journal is to support you to meet your improvement goal, as well as other areas in which your Big Assumptions operate. In the short-term, it is to help guide you so that you gain greater and greater objectivity to your limiting Big Assumption (one dimension of your mindset that currently keeps you from being able to accomplish your health goals).

As you will see, the format of the journal consists of specific reflective process exercises to work on over the next few months. We strongly encourage you pick up each one only as you are ready, and as the book instructs you to. Give yourself time to reflect carefully and deeply on each one – they ***aren't*** a checklist to complete as quickly as you can. Changing your mind takes time and concerted effort. This is your opportunity to apply the ideas to your personal situation, your own mind, your own behavior. As we explain in the introduction, a bridge to take you from where you are to where you want to be doesn't get you anywhere if you don't walk over it.

This journal provides the structure for you to take that walk yourself. Make the journal your own by writing directly into it or using it as a guide —whatever will work best for you!

Here is where your walk toward improved health will take you:

1. **Immunity to Change Map**
   Diagnose your own immunity to change to see what has been holding you back from realizing your improvement goal.

2. **Observing The Big Assumption in Action & Observing Counter-Examples of the Big Assumption:**
   Deepen your understanding of your Big Assumption, including when it "runs" you and when it is inaccurate. Draw on the results of these observations to make your ITC map and Picture of Progress more inclusive of what you are learning.

3. **Picture of Progress:**
   Envision what full success looks like in achieving your improvement goal as you imagine no longer being captive of your Big Assumption.

4. **The Biography of the Big Assumption:**
   When did it get started? What is its history? Reflect on the current relevance of your Big Assumption by understanding when, where and how it originated. By looking back with your current capabilities as an adult on the origin of your Big Assumption, you may develop a more objective relationship to your Big Assumption.

5. **Testing the Big Assumption:**
   Intentionally behave counter to how your Big Assumption would have you act, see what happens, and then reflect on what those results tell you about the certainty of your Big Assumption. Make additions or changes to your ITC map and Picture of Progress based on what you are learning. Test your Big Assumption once, twice, three times or as many times as you need until you are confident of when, if at all, it applies.

6. **Taking Stock:**
   Assess the current status of your Big Assumption, how to maintain your progress, and how to guard against future slippage.

1

Immunity to Change Map

A powerful map is a diagnosis, providing a snapshot picture of what your immunity to change looks like, including what the basic Big Assumptions are that give rise to your immunities. Your map should feel compelling to you. You should be able to see how you have one foot on the gas and one on the brake at the same time.

My Improvement Goal	"Doing and Not Doing"	Hidden Completing Commitments	My Big Assumptions

CHANGE JOURNAL

2

Observing the Big Assumption in Action & Natural Challenges to the Big Assumption

What happens, and fails to happen, as a result of holding your Big Assumption as true? Keep track of situations where you can see (or have recently seen) your Big Assumption at work—e.g., influencing how you look at things, feel about things, take action (or not take action), make choices, spend your energies, etc. These situations may be so abundant that it will make sense for you just to keep track of the several most salient instances. Or, there may only be a few such situations that occur. Feel free to confine your observations to one part of your life (such as just when you are with family, or just with friends) or make note of wherever you see your Big Assumption influencing you.

Directions:

1. Choose one Big Assumption to focus on. Look at your list of Big Assumptions. Are there one or two that feel like they are the most powerful for you? One that is holding you back the most?

2. For the next two weeks, do not attempt to change your behavior or your Big Assumption. Do attend to its influence in your life. Specifically: What do you notice does or does not happen as a result of holding your Big Assumption as TRUE? Write two things down: 1) what happened (including inside of you, what you were thinking and feeling), and 2) what costs did you incur?

The Big Assumption I will focus on:

Describe situation where Big Assumption got in your way (including your thoughts and feelings)	When it got in your way, what specific problems or negative results did your Big Assumption cause you?
Situation #1:	Situation #1:
Situation #2:	Situation #2:
Situation #3:	Situation #3:
Situation #4:	Situation #4:
Situation #5:	Situation #5:

Once you have a few examples of seeing your Big Assumption in action (three or more), you can start to look for patterns and themes. Take a look across all your examples and ask yourself the following kinds of questions:

Observing the Big Assumption in Action: Reflection

What stands out to you? What do you notice most of all?

What thoughts, feelings, perspectives, actions, and choices do you experience when you listen to your B.A.?

Do you see patterns i.e., are there particular types of people, content areas, circumstances (inside yourself or in the environment) that activate your Big Assumption?

Do you notice any additional Big Assumptions you are making? If so, add these to your 4-column map.

Observing Naturally Occurring Counters to the Big Assumption

In addition to looking for examples of your Big Assumption in action, we invite you to be on the lookout for experiences that lead you to question the truthfulness or widespread applicability of your Big Assumption. Because of the "certainty" quality of our Big Assumptions (our difficulty in considering how things could be any "other" than this), our Big Assumptions actually inform what we see and how we see the world. They lead us to attend systematically to certain data and to systematically avoid or ignore other data.

Directions: Actively search for data and experiences—in your professional or personal life—that would counter or cast doubt on the absolute quality of your Big Assumption. Take notes about specific situations, interactions, feelings, etc. *Do not intentionally change anything you do or think relative to your Big Assumption, only take account of any spontaneously occurring experiences that might cast doubt on their absolute quality.* Explain how you see the situation and what happened as potential evidence that your Big Assumption is not 100% accurate.

Describe the situations that challenge your Big Assumption (including your thoughts & feelings)	How could what happened possibly suggest a way that your Big Assumption is wrong or distorted?
Counter Observation #1:	**Counter Observation #1:**
Counter Observation #2:	**Counter Observation #2:**
Counter Observation #3:	**Counter Observation #3:**
Counter Observation #4:	**Counter Observation #4:**

Once you have at least three observations of challenges and counters to your Big Assumption, it's time to step back to see what you can learn from these about your Big Assumption and your mindset, more generally. Take a look across all your examples and ask yourself the following questions:

Observing Counter-Examples of the Big Assumption: Reflection

What stands out to you? What do you notice most of all?

What thoughts, feelings, perspectives, actions, and choices did you experience in these instances?

Do you see any patterns? Is the same doubt about your Big Assumption raised across the different instances? Is there anything in common across the examples that might account for the counter-data? (e.g., particular types of people, content areas, circumstances, inside yourself or in the environment).

Did you act differently than your Big Assumption would have you act? If so, what did you do? What are your hunches about why you acted differently? Was it because of something "out there," or something you said to yourself, or some combination of the two, or anything else?

What does the counter-data suggest to you about your Big Assumption?

What are your key take-aways?

3
Picture of Progress

This exercise is designed to help you plan for your success in meeting your Col. 1 Improvement Goal. Its purpose is to have you envision what success looks like, both short-term and long-term, in terms of how you *think, feel* and *act*, while drawing on your insights into your immune system. The main focus here is on *you*, and your increasing effectiveness in meeting your goal. To be clear, the purpose of identifying these progress steps is NOT to begin immediately trying to accomplish them. The whole point of the immune system concept is that change is not a straight-forward matter as people often think. It may be useful to periodically review and revise your Picture of Progress as you discover new thoughts and feelings through later exercises.

Why we invite you to create this personalized picture of emerging success:

- ✓ A clear picture of success **provides direction**. You are more likely to get where you want to go the more you know where you want to go.
- ✓ Being able to visualize what full success looks like—like athletes do—also **increases the likelihood of being successful** as you imagine effectively engaging in targeted new mindsets & behaviors. This often **releases energy and optimism for improvement**, important allies for personal change.
- ✓ You can safely explore **how revising your Big Assumption can lead to new mindset & behavior options**. In doing so, you may develop potential ways you want to test your Big Assumption.
- ✓ You can use your success picture to **identify what you may need to learn** to be successful. In this way, you plan for success.
- ✓ A completed Picture of Progress **provides a realistic image of the pace of improvement**. Lasting change depends on small, incremental steps, taken over time, with success building upon success.

Directions: *Review your 4-column map before you start this exercise to remind yourself of your immune system and Big Assumption(s).*

1. In the far left column, enter your Column 1 Improvement Goal and Big Assumption(s) that most get in your way.

2. Move to the last column, envisioning "Success": What would it look like if you were to be fully successful in realizing your Column 1 Improvement Goal? **Allow yourself to imagine you are freer of your Big Assumption as you do this.** *Be as specific as you can* along three dimensions: what would you be thinking? Feeling? Doing?

3. (Work backwards from there). What would constitute "significant progress" in moving towards that success? What would enable you to realize more of your Column 1 goal? Again, imagine you are freer of your Big Assumption as you develop this picture of your new thoughts, feelings and actions. Consider incorporating ways you can catch yourself when you are falling into your default mode and get you back on track. Enter your answer in the column entitled, "Significant Progress."

4. Then answer the question, "What first steps will move you forward towards your picture of success?" It is often helpful early in a change process to tell at least one person about your intentions. Consider whether there is someone you want to talk with and even ask for his or her support. Enter your answers in the column entitled, "1st Steps Forward."

Picture of Progress Overview

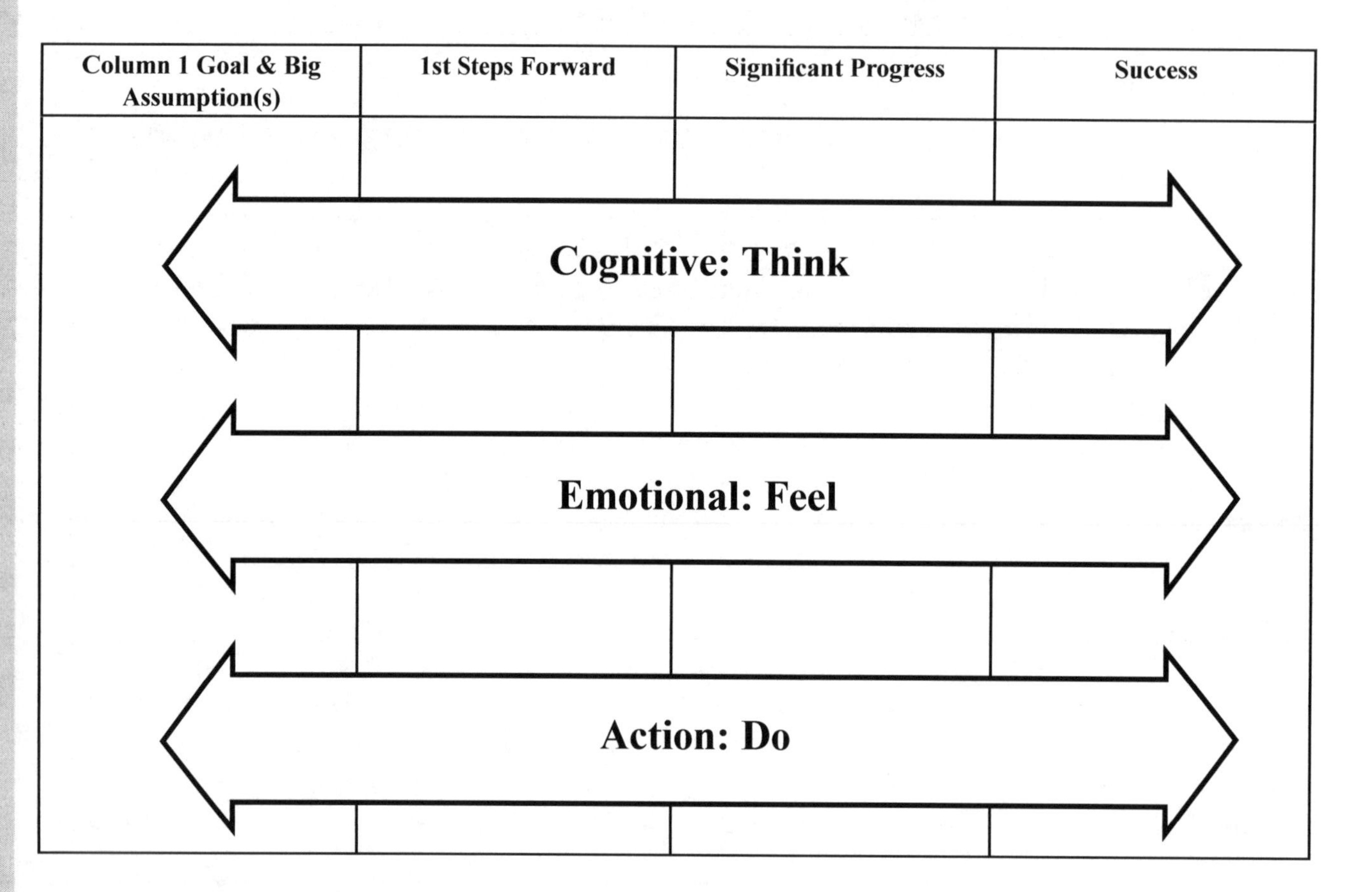

Your Picture of Progress Should:

- Focus on you (not others)
- Incorporate the what *and* the how of new behaviors
- Generate potential future ideas for testing your Big Assumption
- Relate beyond adaptive requirements to technical ones, where needed
- Connect to your Big Assumption

Your Picture of Progress:

Column 1 Goal & Big Assumption(s)	1st Steps Forward	Significant Progress	Success

C H A N G E J O U R N A L

4

Charting the Biography of Your Big Assumption: Approach #1

Directions: Thinking back over the first 15 or 16 years of life, identify a handful memories that continue to stick with you and that were in some way negative (disturbing, puzzling, made you angry, upsetting, scary) in quality. They don't have to be events that were momentous – include events that may now seem tiny, mundane, common for many young people to experience in their lives. If these events were called up for you in your reflection, include them in your list. Record these events in column one below and fill out the rest of the table accordingly

Events (the headlines)	What I was thinking at that time	What I was feeling at that time	Lessons learned/ conclusions drawn at that time

Question 2: What connections, if any, do you make between the fourth column on your Biography Chart and the fourth column on your ITC map? Write your responses in the space provided.

In what ways does the biography (or biographic moment) explain your Big Assumption?

Does your biography (or biographic moment) illuminate any additional Big Assumptions you might be making? Do you notice any definitive, i.e., this- always-happens, quality?

To what extent do you believe and feel the situation or events from your biography (or biographic moment) apply to your current life? If you think they do, how so?

Charting the Biography of the Big Assumption: Approach #2

Directions: What is the "history" of your Big Assumption? When was it born? Are there specific situations, feelings, important events or moments you can recall? How long has your BA been around? What were some of its critical turning points? Perhaps there is one story, event, snapshot, or episode that captures something from your past that may have gotten your Big Assumption started or served to emphasize its importance. ***Again, do not intentionally change anything you do or think relative to your Big Assumption.*** Enter your response below.

Here are a few questions you might find useful:

In what ways does the biography (or biographic moment) explain your Big Assumption?

Does your biography (or biographic moment) illuminate any additional Big Assumptions you might be making? Do you notice any definitive, “this-always-happens” quality?

To what extent do you believe and feel the situation or events from your biography (or biographic moment) apply to your current life? If you think they do, how so?

5
Designing a Test of Your Big Assumption

Testing Big Assumptions is at the heart of overturning an immunity to change. *The purpose of a test is to see what happens when you intentionally alter your usual behavior in order to learn about the accuracy of your Big Assumption.* (In other words, the purpose of a test is to "get information" not immediately to improve or "get better.") Everything you have been doing up until now is to better prepare you to design, run and make sense of the results of testing your Big Assumption.

The goal of this exercise is for you to design a test of one of your Big Assumptions. It is <u>preparation</u> for actually running your first "formal" test.

A good test meets **S-M-A-R-T** criteria:

1) **S-M:** it is important that your experiment be both **safe** and **modest**. Safe means that if the worst case outcome were to occur, you could live with it! Modest means that you can the test is relatively easy to carry out (ideally, it doesn't require you to go out of your way at all, but rather is an opportunity to do something different in your normal day). It can also mean you make a *small* change in what you do.

2) **A:** a good test will be **actionable** in the near-term. This means that you are able to carry it out within the next week or so. You can easily imagine a setting or upcoming situation in which to run your test.

3) **R-T:** finally, a good test **researches** the question, "how accurate is my Big Assumption?" and, like any good research, it requires collecting data (including data that would qualify your assumption or call it into doubt). In addition to how people react to you, *your feelings* can be a very rich data source. The test, in fact, **tests** your Big Assumption. A "test" should not be some clever way to prove that your Big Assumption is true! Your test should be designed so that it can generate disconfirming data, if it exists.

Designing Your First Test

Directions:

Option 1: Start with the end in mind: what *data* would lead you to doubt your Big Assumption? (If you can't imagine what data could challenge or cast doubt on your assumption, then you don't have a testable assumption.) Work backwards from there to figure out what action you could take that could generate that data.

Option 2: What *behavior* you could change (start or stop doing) that would get you useful information about the accuracy of your Big Assumption? Here are some options from which to choose:

- Alter a behavior from your Column 2
- Perform an action that runs counter to your Column 3 Hidden Commitment
- Start directly from your Big Assumption (Column 4): "What experiment would give me information (as to whether, e.g., the if-then sequence built into the assumption is really so certain)?"
- Go to your Picture of Progress and enact a version of a next recognizable step
- Go to your Observations of Counters to your Big Assumption and try an intentional version of one of these

Whichever option you choose, design your test so that *it meets the S-M-A-R-T criteria.*

CHANGE JOURNAL

My Big Assumption Says:	So I will (Change my Behavior This Way)…	And collect the following data …	In Order to Find Out Whether …
		• Is there anyone to whom you'd like to give a "heads-up" or ask to serve as an observer who can give you feedback after the fact?	

Review your test on these criteria:	Yes	Not Sure
Is it safe? (If the worst case were to happen, you could live with the results).		
Is the data relevant to your Big Assumption?		
Does it have face-validity? (The test actually tests your Big Assumption)		
Are the data sources valid? (No one is either out to get you or wants to protect or save you).		
Might it "re-true" your Big Assumption? (Is it designed so that it surely will lead to bad consequences, just as your BA tells you? Are you setting yourself up to fail? Is there any data you could collect that could disconfirm your BA?)		
Is it actionable in the near-term? (e.g., the people or situation you need in order to enact the test are available, you are reasonably certain you know how to do what you plan, and you can run the test within the next week or so).		

Running and Interpreting Your Test

Designing an effective test of your Big Assumption is one step. Running it is a next step. Now is the time to look at your data for the sole purpose of understanding what it suggests about your Big Assumption. **Remember, the purpose of running a good test is not to see whether you improved, i.e., whether your behavior change "worked" (although this is not unimportant!), but rather to use the test results to inform your Big Assumption.** You will know you are on track with this exercise if you can see what aspect of your Big Assumption, if any, is confirmed by the data, and what aspect, if any, is disconfirmed.

Here are a few tips to keep in mind when you interpret your data:

- ➜ The point of a test is not to outright reject a Big Assumption, but rather to help sharpen its contours so you have a realistic, data-based version of when, where and with whom your Big Assumption is relevant. (Even relatively modest changes to a Big Assumption can overturn an immunity to change.)

- ➜ No one experiment is likely to be conclusive about a Big Assumption.

- ➜ When our Big Assumptions have a powerful hold on us, they direct us to predictable interpretations—ones that keep the Big Assumption alive and well! An antidote to this tendency is to push yourself to generate at least one additional interpretation of the data. (If nothing comes to mind, then try this: Imagine you are someone else, a real person, who happened to be in that exact situation, and the same things happened. How would this person make sense of what happened? If that doesn't get you anywhere, then find a person you trust to offer his or her interpretation.)

Directions:

1. Write your Big Assumption below.

2. Then write what you *actually* did to test your Big Assumption; this may be what you planned to do (in which case, you can simply copy the text from your test design), or you may have done something else (which is fine!).

3. Write what you observed happening. This includes what you saw and heard other people do or say, as well as what you were feeling.

4. Write what you learned about the accuracy of your Big Assumption

My Big Assumption says:

So in order to test it I changed my behavior this way:

This is what I observed happening:

And this is what the data tells me about my Big Assumption:

Remember that no one test is likely to be conclusive about a Big Assumption. Often, the second and third tests are versions of the first one. What differs is the person, circumstance or level of risk. It is the cumulative weight of several tests that, in most cases, begins to overturn the person's Immunity to Change—the whole purpose of these exercises. Once the Big Assumption no longer has its force, the self-protective Column 3 Commitment is no longer necessary and we stop needing to generate the obstructive Column 2 behaviors.

Designing Your Second Test

Directions: What are your thoughts about a next test of your Big Assumption? Pick up on what you've learned about your Big Assumption. What next test could you design to learn more?

This may also be a good time to revisit your Picture of Progress to check whether it reflects any new thoughts, feelings and behaviors you have access to now that you have begun to formally test your Big Assumption.

CHANGE JOURNAL

My Big Assumption Says:	So I will (Change my Behavior This Way)…	And collect the following data …	In Order to Find Out Whether …
		• Is there anyone to whom you'd like to give a "heads-up" or ask to serve as an observer who can give you feedback after the fact?	

Review your test on these criteria:	Yes	Not Sure
Is it safe? (If the worst case were to happen, you could live with the results).		
Is the data relevant to your Big Assumption?		
Does it have face-validity? (The test actually tests your Big Assumption)		
Are the data sources valid? (No one is either out to get you or wants to protect or save you).		
Might it "re-true" your Big Assumption? (Is it designed so that it surely will lead to bad consequences, just as your BA tells you? Are you setting yourself up to fail? Is there any data you could collect that could disconfirm your BA?)		
Is it actionable in the near-term? (e.g., the people or situation you need in order to enact the test are available, you are reasonably certain you know how to do what you plan, and you can run the test within the next week or so).		

A quick reminder of a few tips to keep in mind when you interpret your data:

- ✓ Can you see contours of your Big Assumption, i.e., "when, where and with whom" it is and is not relevant?
- ✓ No one experiment is likely to be conclusive about a Big Assumption.
- ✓ Can you generate at least one additional interpretation of the data?

CHANGE JOURNAL

Second Test Reflection: What happened and how you make sense of it:

My Big Assumption says:

So in order to test it I changed my behavior this way:

This is what I observed happening:

And this is what the data tells me about my Big Assumption:

Designing Your Third Test

My Big Assumption Says:	So I will (Change my Behavior This Way)...	And collect the following data ...	In Order to Find Out Whether ...
		• Is there anyone to whom you'd like to give a "heads-up" or ask to serve as an observer who can give you feedback after the fact?	

CHANGE JOURNAL

Review your test on these criteria:	**Yes**	**Not Sure**
Is it safe? (If the worst case were to happen, you could live with the results).		
Is the data relevant to your Big Assumption?		
Does it have face-validity? (The test actually tests your Big Assumption)		
Are the data sources valid? (No one is either out to get you or wants to protect or save you).		
Might it "re-true" your Big Assumption? (Is it designed so that it surely will lead to bad consequences, just as your BA tells you? Are you setting yourself up to fail? Is there any data you could collect that could disconfirm your BA?)		
Is it actionable in the near-term? (e.g., the people or situation you need in order to enact the test are available, you are reasonably certain you know how to do what you plan, and you can run the test within the next week or so).		

A quick reminder of a few tips to keep in mind when you interpret your data:

- ✓ Can you see contours of your Big Assumption, i.e., "when, where and with whom" it is and is not relevant?
- ✓ No one experiment is likely to be conclusive about a Big Assumption.
- ✓ Can you generate at least one additional interpretation of the data?

Third Test Reflection: What happened and how you make sense of it:

My Big Assumption Says:

So in Order to Test it I Changed my Behavior This Way:

This is What I Observed Happening:

And This is What the data Tells me about my Big Assumption:

Feel free to plan and run additional tests. While you are exploring your Big Assumption, you may discover that it would be valuable to test another assumption. That often happens. If so, revisit the test exercises with the new assumption (you might want to do the self-observations exercises first).

6
Taking Stock

You hopefully have seen personal progress towards your improvement goal by this point in the overcoming-immunities process. You may also be wondering, just about now, whether you are going to be able to sustain your good progress. We all have had experiences of slipping back into old habits and patterns, so we can legitimately ask, "Why should this be any different?"

One way to help yourself not slip back is to consolidate your current progress on overcoming your immunity. This exercise is designed to help you do just that. By assessing where you on in the following developmental sequence, you will be able to make informed choices about what next steps will deepen or anchor your new learning.

Development Sequence for Overcoming Immunities to Change

UNCONSCIOUSLY "IMMUNE"

▼

CONSCIOUSLY "IMMUNE"

CONSCIOUSLY "RELEASED"

UNCONSCIOUSLY "RELEASED"

Reflecting on where you are in the process of overcoming your immunity to change:

Take a moment now to think about exactly where you are in overcoming your immunity. To do that, use the following basic descriptions of what it means to be "Consciously Released" and "Unconsciously Released."

"Consciously Released": Testing your Big Assumption(s) and discovering the conditions under which it is and is not valid is a crucial part of this development phase. This may include discovering that the Big Assumption is not warranted in any situation. Often people learn new behaviors and new "self-talk" scripts as a part of this testing process. When you can act on your newly discovered knowledge to interrupt the Big Assumption (and the old behavior and self talk patterns associated with it) in those situations where it is not valid, you are demonstrating the new capacity to be "Consciously Released" from your Big Assumption. This takes mindful practice. The journey is not a bump-free or necessarily straight one. It is normal to fall back into old patterns associated with the Big Assumption. Still, knowing that you're falling back, and knowing how you can get yourself unstuck are all signs of development. You should also see that you have made progress towards meeting your Column 1 goal.

"Unconsciously Released": When you no longer need to stop, think and plan in order to interrupt your Big Assumption, you have developed the capacity to be "Unconsciously Released" from it. At this point, you automatically act and think in ways that run counter to your previously held Big Assumption in those situations where it is not valid. New beliefs and understandings, informed and developed mindfully throughout the process, have taken the place of the Big Assumption. You have likely made significant progress, if not full success, towards meeting your Column 1 goal.

Which of these two descriptions speaks to you?

If your self-assessment is that you are "Unconsciously Released," then this exercise will be a useful summary of your work to date. If "Consciously Released" better describes your current relationship to your Big Assumption, then you may want to continue with further tests of your Big Assumption (a good choice especially if you are aware that your Big Assumption grabs hold of you frequently) and use the results of this exercise to focus those tests. The testing process is iterative and there is no set number of tests that, if done, will overturn an immune system. Keep with testing until you no longer feel hooked by your Big Assumption.

Directions: Review this development sequence and comment on where you see yourself in the sequence at this time. You may find the following questions useful as you take stock of where you are:

Where do you see yourself in the sequence at this time?

Have you reached any conclusions, or have any hunches about conditions under which your Big Assumption is *valid*? Think about particular situations – who, what, where and when.

Have you reached any conclusions, or have any hunches about conditions under which your Big Assumption is *invalid*? Think about particular situations – who, what, where and when

Do you find your Big Assumption asserting itself in situations you know it ought not? If so, do you have any generalizations about the conditions under which you are likely (more or less) to find yourself being sucked into the old patterns associated with the Big Assumption? What still sometimes *hooks* you?

Are there key "releases" (i.e., self-talk that unhooks you) you have developed and can use to help yourself easily and readily when you are facing your Big Assumption in real-time?

To what extent / how often can you use these "releases" to help you from being pulled into old patterns?

Have you developed new behaviors or ways of taking to yourself in situations that used to activate your Big Assumption?

Think about situations in which you think your Big Assumption is no longer accurate. What new beliefs or understandings do you hold about "how things work" or what will happen in these situations?

How would you rate your progress toward achieving your Column 1 goal? Has your understanding of, or relationship to, that goal changed in important ways?

Made in the USA
Middletown, DE
01 April 2016